LOGAN'S
ILLUSTRATED HUMAN ANATOMY

ANATOMY

A PICTORIAL INTRODUCTION TO BASIC FORM AND STRUCTURE

LOGAN'S
ILLUSTRATED HUMAN ANATOMY

A PICTORIAL INTRODUCTION TO BASIC FORM AND STRUCTURE

BARI M. LOGAN MA FMA Hon MBIE MAMAA
Formerly University Prosector, Department of Anatomy,
University of Cambridge; Prosector Department of Anatomy,
Royal College of Surgeons of England, London and Anatomical
Preparator, Department of Human Morphology, University of
Nottingham, Queen's Medical School, UK

Photography by **Adrian Newman**

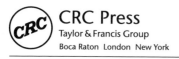
CRC Press
Taylor & Francis Group
Boca Raton London New York

CRC Press is an imprint of the
Taylor & Francis Group, an **informa** business

CRC Press
Taylor & Francis Group
6000 Broken Sound Parkway NW, Suite 300
Boca Raton, FL 33487-2742

© 2017 by Bari M. Logan
CRC Press is an imprint of Taylor & Francis Group, an Informa business

No claim to original U.S. Government works

Printed in the UK by Severn, Gloucester on responsibly sourced paper

Version Date: 20160519

International Standard Book Number-13: 978-1-4987-5530-6 (Pack - Book and Ebook)

Visit the Taylor & Francis Web site at
http://www.taylorandfrancis.com

and the CRC Press Web site at
http://www.crcpress.com

DEDICATION

For

Arlette Herzig and Robert Logan

And

To the memory of an esteemed colleague and true friend

Professor R.M.H. (Bob) McMinn
(1923–2012)

CONTENTS

PART I HEAD, NECK, BRAIN AND UPPER SPINAL CORD

Contents

PART II VERTEBRAL COLUMN, SPINAL CORD, SKELETON AND TRUNK

PART III UPPER LIMB

PART VI LOWER LIMB

APPENDIX

Visit **www.crcpress.com/cw/logan** for:

- A library of all the cadaver images from the book, in labelled and unlabelled versions, for use in presentations and lectures.
- A 'drag-and-drop' self-test in which you can test your ability to identify correctly key anatomical landmarks in the images from the book – ideal during pressured exam revision.

Together, these materials bring additional utility to the beautifully prepared and presented images in the textbook. We hope you find them useful!

FOREWORD

I was delighted to be asked to write this Foreword to *Logan's Illustrated Human Anatomy*. I had the great pleasure to teach for six years in the Department of Anatomy at the University of Cambridge with Bari Logan as my colleague. I was immediately impressed by the exquisite prosections that he executed for our classes, which were of a standard that I had not seen before (or, indeed, since), and which greatly facilitated our teaching. The quality of the material was outstanding as result of the technique devised by Bari to preserve the bodies. It was a joy for me to watch him, with his magnifying glasses perched on his nose, dissecting with the skill of a master. He went on to produce outstanding sections of an entire cadaver in preparing for the *Atlas of Sectional Anatomy* that we later published together.

Bari Logan has published a whole series of anatomical texts and atlases over the years and this, his latest, represents a distillation of his skill. There is no substitute for the study of actual dissection material, osteological specimens and the surface anatomy of the living subject. However, this atlas will provide a valuable teaching aid to surgical trainees, medical students, nurses, physiotherapists and, in fact, all members of the health care professions whose study includes a good working knowledge of anatomy, not just for their examinations but also for their daily work with patients.

To all of them I commend this beautifully prepared atlas.

Professor Harold Ellis CBE, FRCS
Emeritus Professor of Surgery, University of London, London, UK
Clinical Anatomist, Guy's Campus, University of London, London, UK

PREFACE

Welcome to *Logan's Illustrated Human Anatomy*, a picture book intended to widen or test the anatomical knowledge of the reader through keen observation.

It has been said that human anatomy is a difficult subject to learn and an easy subject to forget and this comment I certainly found to be true during the early years of my career as an anatomical preparator in the late 1970s.

However, through hours of meticulous dissection work and continual reference to many illustrated texts, I soon developed a clear understanding of how the human frame is constructed.

Some 40 years on, herewith is my contribution to the library, which contains what I consider to be some of the best examples of my dissection work done between the years 1980 to 2003; in addition, a few from colleagues are included that are well worthy of publication, for appreciation by the discerning student.

Most of the pictures offer standard views of anatomy that one should expect to encounter when studying specimens in any medical school dissecting room or museum; a few offer novel views of structures in greater detail and these should enhance the norm and hopefully delight and challenge the knowledgeable.

A few pictures of bones have been included in each section of the book, some not labelled in great detail, but there to help the reader to try to visualise the internal supporting skeleton in relation to surrounding soft tissue structures. The in-depth study of human osteology is a discipline in its own right and there are many detailed illustrated texts on the subject, as are commercially available accurate life-size replica bones, which offer the advantage, to be encouraged, of home study away from the dissecting room.

I hope that this book of human anatomy pictures will stimulate interest in the subject, be appreciated by students and professional practitioners alike and become a valued addition to any medical bookshelf, thus adding another 'tiny cog' to the great wheel of medical education.

Bari M. Logan
Siegershausen, Switzerland, April 2016

ACKNOWLEDGEMENTS

The author is most grateful to the following:

For photography, digital expertise and advice: Mr Adrian Newman, Mr Ian Bolton and Mr John Bashford.

Original skeleton artwork: Mrs Rachael Chesterton.

All of the Anatomy Audio Visual Group (AVMG), Department of Physiology, Development and Neuroscience, University of Cambridge, UK.

For expert anatomical advice over the years with picture annotations: Mr Clive Brewis, Mr David Chapireau, Prof Adrian Dixon, Prof Harold Ellis, Mr Ralph Hutchings, Mr Mark McCarthy, Prof 'Bob' McMinn, Dr Catherine Molyneux, Prof Ian Parkin, Prof Pat Reynolds, Mr Dishan Singh, Mr Robert Whitaker.

The majority of the illustrations used are reproduced with permission from:

Core Anatomy Illustrated, I.Parkin, B.M. Logan and M. McCarthy (Hodder Arnold 2007).

And some from:

Human Sectional Anatomy – Atlas of Body Sections, CT and MRI Images, 4th edition, H. Ellis, B.M. Logan, A.K. Dixon and D.J. Bowden (CRC Press, 2015).

McMinn's Colour Atlas of Head and Neck Anatomy, 4th edition, B.M. Logan, P.A. Reynolds and R.T. Hutchings (Mosby Elsevier, 2010).

McMinn's Colour Atlas of Foot and Ankle Anatomy, 4th edition, B.M. Logan, R.T. Hutchings (Elsevier Saunders, 2012).

'Muscles of the body' is reproduced with permission from *McMinn's Functional and Clinical Anatomy*, R.M.H. McMinn, P. Gaddum-Rosse, R.T. Hutchings and B.M. Logan (Mosby-Wolfe, 1995).

The author would like to thank Joanna Koster and Paul Bennett, and the team at CRC Press, for their help, advice and support.

AND A SPECIAL THANKS

The author wishes to express his most profound gratitude to those who bequeathed their bodies to medical science and also to their loved ones and close relatives for supporting those wishes.

Without these important selfless donations, the discipline of human anatomy could not be taught at both preclinical and postgraduate level to the detailed high standard of knowledge essential to the practice of good medicine.

ABOUT THE AUTHOR

Bari Logan has 33 years practical experience in the preparation of human anatomical material for both preclinical and postgraduate medical studies, museum display and research with direct clinical relevance.

He began his career as Anatomical Preparator in 1972 at Nottingham University in the newly developing Queen's Medical School; then in 1977 moved to London where he took-up the academic post of Prosector to the Department of Anatomy, Royal College of Surgeons, of England under the Professorship of R.M.H. McMinn.

A final career move, in 1987, took him to the University of Cambridge, as University Prosector to the Anatomy Department, where part of his duties was to re-develop and oversee the day-to-day running of a busy undergraduate dissecting room facility; he retired in 2005.

He has co-authored nine major books on the subject of Human Anatomy which have produced over 60 foreign editions in 17 different languages.

During his career he has gained numerous professional qualifications and awards in recognition for his work and was elected a member of Clare College Cambridge in 1995.

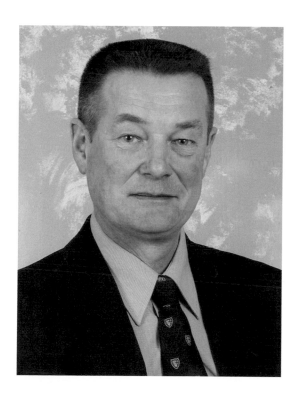

ANATOMICAL PREPARATION CREDITS

The following individuals are credited for their many hours of skilled and meticulous work in the art of preparing the anatomical material illustrated:

Mrs Carmen Bester 161, 169

Dr Neil Borley 31

Ms Mel Lazenby 120, 121, 147

Bari M. Logan 5, 7, 8, 9, 10, 11, 12, 13, 14, 15, 18, 19, 20, 21, 22, 23, 24, 25, 26, 27, 28, 29, 30, 32, 33, 34, 35, 36, 37, 38, 39A, 39B, 40A, 40B, 41, 44A, 44B, 45, 46A, 46B, 47A, 47B, 48A, 48B, 49A, 49B, 49C, 51, 52A, 52B, 53, 54, 55, 56, 57, 58A, 58B, 59, 60A, 61B, 62, 64, 68, 69, 71, 73, 77, 80, 81, 82, 86, 90, 91, 92, 93, 94, 95, 101, 102, 103, 104, 105, 106, 107, 108, 109, 110, 111, 112, 113, 114, 115, 116, 117, 118, 119, 125, 126, 127, 128, 129, 130, 131, 133, 134, 135, 136, 137A, 138B, 139, 131A, 131B, 141, 144, 145, 146, 151, 152, 153, 154, 155, 156, 157, 158, 160, 162, 166, 167

Ms Lynette Nearn 163

Mr Martin Watson 168

Ms Lucy Whitehead 79, 84, 85, 87

Messrs Adam, Rouilly UK Ltd (Osteological Material) 2A, 2B, 3, 4, 5, 6, 7, 16, 17, 42, 43, 50, 51, 58C, 61, 65, 66A, 66B, 66C, 67A, 67B, 70, 72, 76A, 76B, 83A, 83B, 88, 89, 98, 99, 100, 124, 142, 143, 150A, 150B, 159A, 159B, 164, 165

INTRODUCTION

CURRENT TERMINOLOGY

Terminology used conforms to the International Anatomical Terminology – *Terminology Anatomica* created in 1998 by the Federative Committee on Anatomical Terminology (FCAT) and approved by the 56 member Associations of the International Federation of Associations of Anatomists. (IFAA ISBN 3 –13-115251-6 [book and CD-ROM].)

ROMAN NUMERALS

It is worth noting that Roman numerals are often used when numbering the following anatomical structures, some by long tradition and some (segments) more recently for specific diagnostic and/or surgical intervention purposes.

Cranial nerves –   I–XII

Cervical vertebrae –   CI–CVII

Thoracic vertebrae –   TI–TXII

Lumbar vertebrae –   LI–LV

Sacrum – sacral vertebrae –   I–V

Coccyx – coccygeal vertebrae –   I–IV

Ribs –   I–XII

Metacarpal bones –   I–V

Metatarsal bones –   I–V

Toes –   I–V

Segments of the lungs –   Left: SI–SX; Right: SI–SX

Segments of the bronchi –   Left: BI + BII; Right: BI–BX

Segments of the liver –   I–VIII

For reference:			
1 – I	6 – VI	11 – XI	16 – XVI
2 – II	7 – VII	12 – XII	17 – XVII
3 – III	8 – VIII	13 – XIII	18 – XVIII
4 – IV	9 – IX	14 – XIV	19 – XIX
5 – V	10 – X	15 – XV	20 – XX

OBSERVING THE BODY – GENERAL PARTS

Anterior view

Body standing erect in correct anatomical position with the right forearm in supination (palm of hand facing forwards) and left arm not in anatomical position (tucked to side).

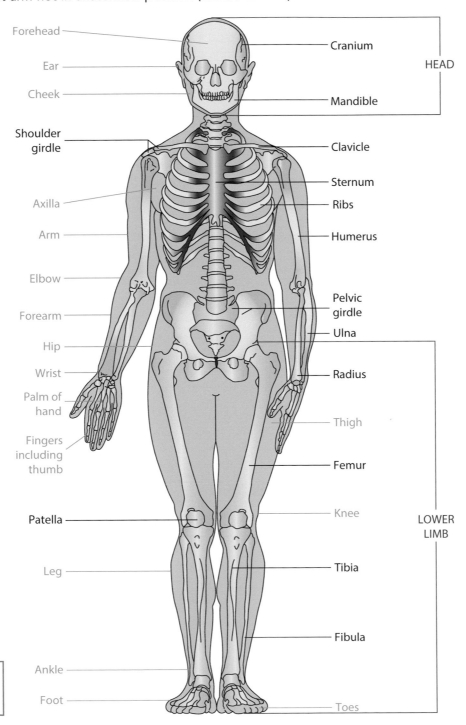

Forehead — Cranium

HEAD

Ear —

Cheek — Mandible

Shoulder girdle — Clavicle

Sternum

Axilla — Ribs

Arm — Humerus

Elbow —

Forearm — Pelvic girdle

Hip — Ulna

Wrist —

Palm of hand — Radius

Fingers including thumb — Thigh

Femur

Patella — Knee

LOWER LIMB

Leg — Tibia

Fibula

Ankle —

Foot — Toes

S
R — L
I

Posterior view

Body standing erect in correct anatomical position with the right forearm in supination (palm of hand facing forwards) and left arm not in anatomical position (tucked to side).

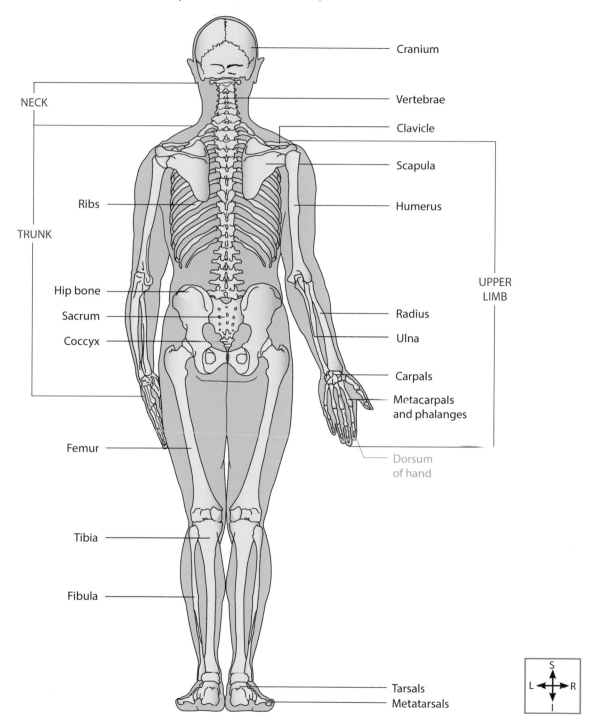

NECK

TRUNK

Ribs

Hip bone

Sacrum

Coccyx

Femur

Tibia

Fibula

Cranium

Vertebrae

Clavicle

Scapula

Humerus

UPPER
LIMB

Radius

Ulna

Carpals

Metacarpals
and phalanges

Dorsum
of hand

Tarsals
Metatarsals

Lateral view

Body standing erect in correct anatomical position, but with the left arm to side and forearm pronated (palm of hand facing backwards).

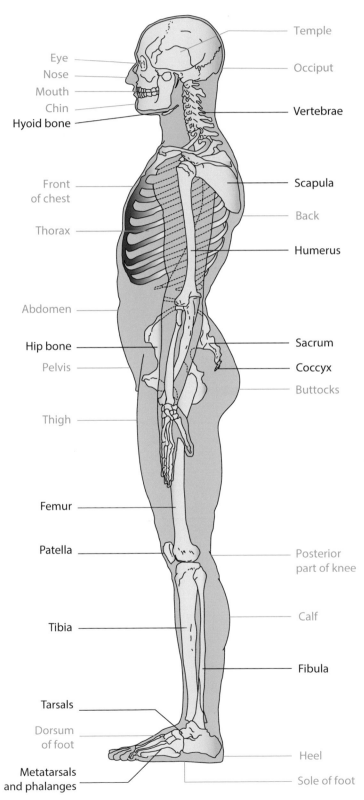

Temple

Eye

Nose

Mouth

Chin

Hyoid bone

Occiput

Vertebrae

Front of chest

Thorax

Scapula

Back

Humerus

Abdomen

Hip bone

Pelvis

Thigh

Sacrum

Coccyx

Buttocks

Femur

Patella

Tibia

Posterior part of knee

Calf

Fibula

Tarsals

Dorsum of foot

Metatarsals and phalanges

Heel

Sole of foot

PLANES OF SECTION

Median sagittal plane

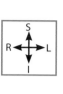

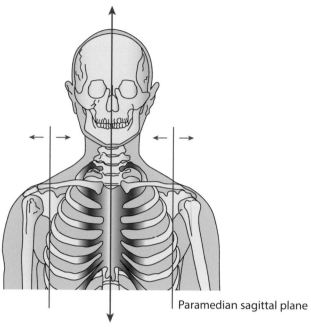

Paramedian sagittal plane

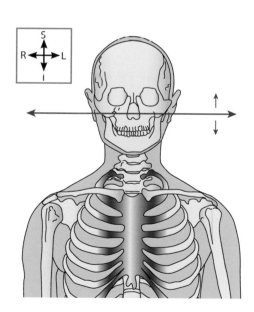

Transverse (axial) plane

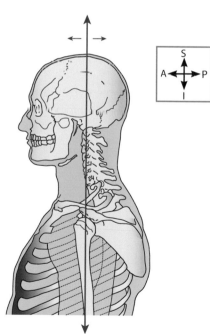

Coronal (frontal) plane

MOVEMENTS OF THE BODY

Abduction: movement away from the midline of the body.

Adduction: movement toward the midline of the body.

Eversion: turning outward.

Inversion: turning inward.

Flexion: bending.

Extension: extending or stretching, straightening out.

Pronation: twisting or turning bones over one another.

Supination: untwisting bones over one another.
   (Pronation and supination are terms specific to the forearm bones, radius and ulna.)

Rotation: twisting in the long axis of a bone.

Shoulder and upper limb

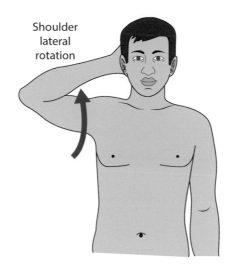

Shoulder lateral rotation

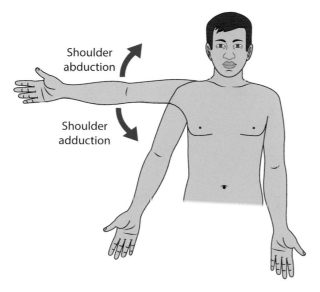

Shoulder abduction

Shoulder adduction

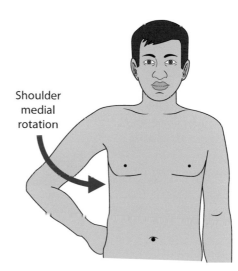

Shoulder medial rotation

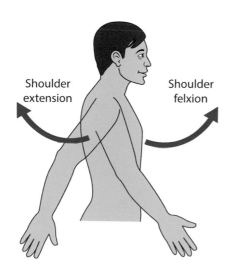

Shoulder extension

Shoulder felxion

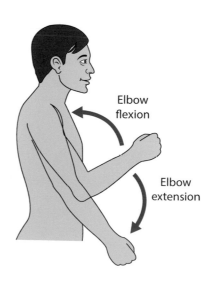

Elbow flexion

Elbow extension

Forearm, wrist and hand

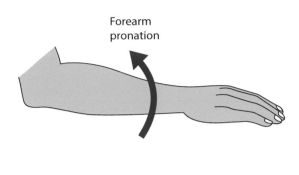

Forearm
pronation

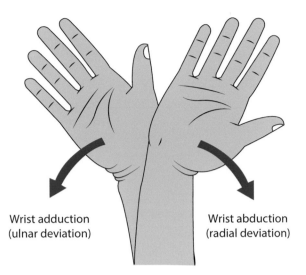

Wrist adduction
(ulnar deviation)

Wrist abduction
(radial deviation)

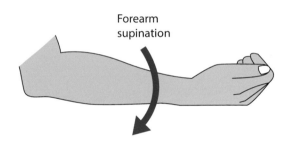

Forearm
supination

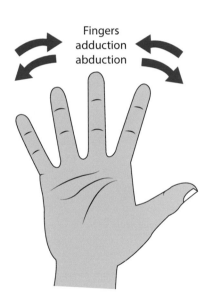

Fingers
adduction
abduction

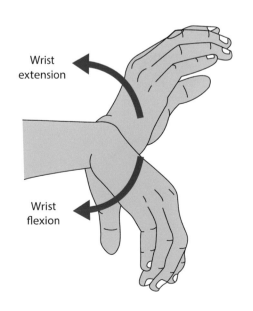

Wrist
extension

Wrist
flexion

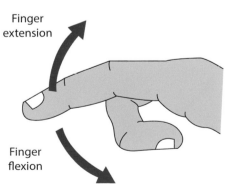

Finger
extension

Finger
flexion

Trunk and lower limb

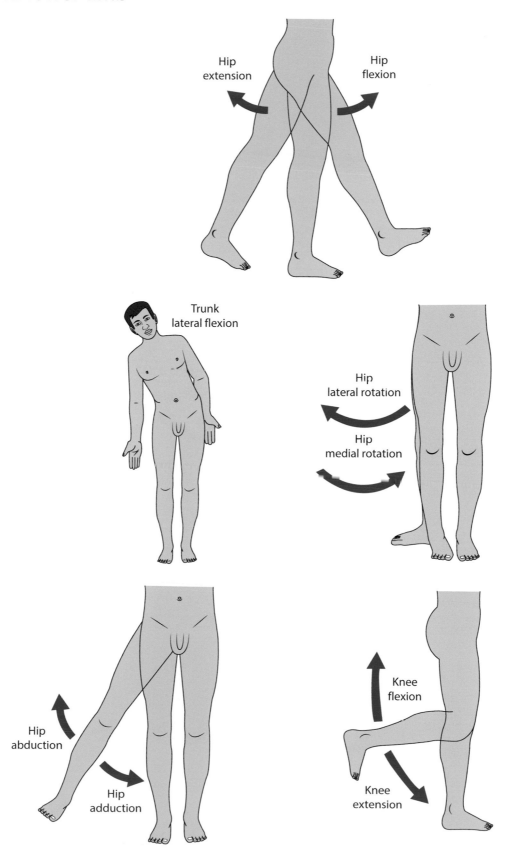

Hip
extension

Hip
flexion

Trunk
lateral flexion

Hip
lateral rotation

Hip
medial rotation

Hip
abduction

Hip
adduction

Knee
flexion

Knee
extension

Ankle and foot

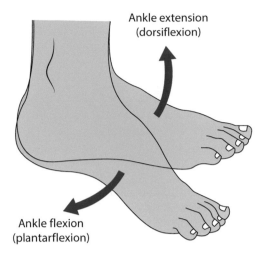

Ankle extension
(dorsiflexion)

Ankle flexion
(plantarflexion)

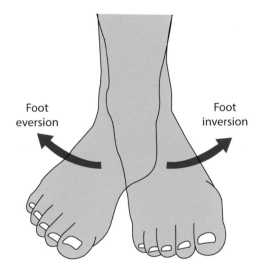

Foot
eversion

Foot
inversion

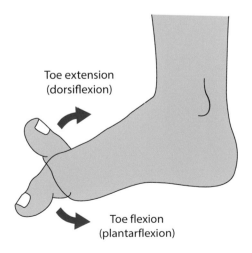

Toe extension
(dorsiflexion)

Toe flexion
(plantarflexion)

ORIENTATION GUIDES

Orientation guides appear with each illustration abbreviated as:

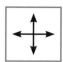

S – superior;   **I** – inferior.

R – right;   **L** – left.

A – anterior;   **P** – posterior.

M – medial;   **L** – lateral.

Limbs: **Prox** – proximal and **Dis** – distal.

Dor – dorsal.

Palm of hand: **Pal** – palmar.

Sole of foot: **Plan** – plantar.

PRESERVATION OF CADAVERS – TECHNICAL INFORMATION

The long-term preservation of cadavers utilised for anatomical dissections (prosections) and preparations illustrated in this book, was by standard embalming technique, using an electric motor pump set at a constant pressure rate of 15 psi (1.06 Bar).

Perfusion of tissues was achieved through the arterial system via femoral artery cannulation of one leg and return drainage of the accompanying vein. On the acceptance of 25 litres of preservative fluid by pump, local injection of those areas not visibly affected was carried out by automatic syringe. On average 30 litres of preservative fluid was used to preserve each cadaver, variable according to size.

Immediately following the embalming process, cadavers were encapsulated in thick gauge clear polythene bags and cold stored at a temperature of 10.6°C (51°F) at a 40% humidity rating for a minimum period of 16 weeks before dissection. This period of storage allowed the preservative fluid to saturate the body tissues thoroughly, resulting in a highly satisfactory state of preservation.

The chemical formula for 20 litres of preservative fluid (Logan *et al.*, 1989) is:

Methylated spirit 64 over proof	12.5 litres
Phenol liquefied 80%	2.5 litres
Formaldehyde solution 38%	1.5 litres
Glycerine BP	3.5 litres

The resultant working strength and basic action of each constituent is:

Methylated spirit	55% – fixative and preservative
Glycerine	12% – preservative and plasticiser
Phenol	10% – antiseptic and disinfectant
Formaldehyde solution	3% – fixative

The advantages of using this particular preservative fluid are:

- A state of soft preservation is achieved, benefiting dissection techniques.
- The low formaldehyde solution content obviates excessive noxious fumes during dissection.
- A degree of natural tissue colour is maintained, benefitting photography.
- Mould growth does not occur on either whole cadavers thus preserved or their subsequent dissected (prosected) and stored parts.

Safety footnote

Since the preparation of the anatomical material illustrated in this book, there have been substantial changes to health and safety regulations concerning the handling and use of certain chemical constituents in preservative (embalming) fluids. It is essential therefore, to seek official local health and safety advice and guidance if intending to adopt the above preservative fluid.

PART I

Head, Neck, Brain and Upper Spinal Cord

Skull of full-term fetus – *A from the front; B from above*

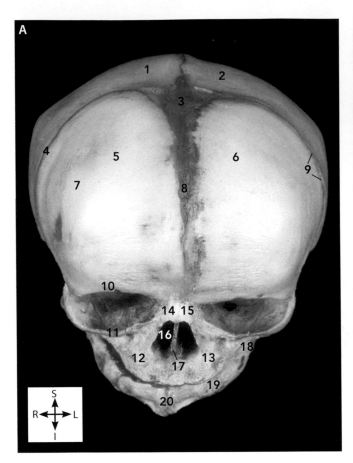

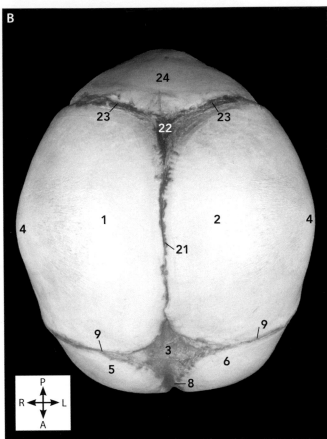

1	Right	} parietal bone	9	Coronal suture	17	Nasal septum
2	Left		10	Supra-orbital margin	18	Ramus } of mandible
3	Anterior fontanelle		11	Infra-orbital margin	19	Body
4	Parietal tuberosity		12	Right } maxilla	20	Symphysis menti
5	Right	} frontal bone	13	Left	21	Sagittal suture
6	Left		14	Right } nasal bone	22	Posterior fontanelle
7	Frontal tuberosity		15	Left	23	Lambdoid suture
8	Frontal (metopic) suture		16	Anterior nasal aperture	24	Occipital bone

Skull of full-term fetus – *C from the left*

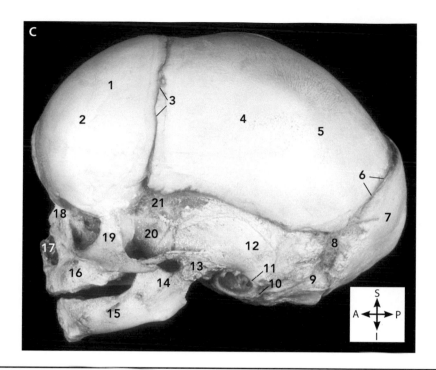

1 Left frontal bone	9 Petrous part of temporal bone	16 Maxilla
2 Frontal tuberosity	10 Stylomastoid foramen	17 Septal cartilage
3 Coronal suture	11 Tympanic ring	18 Nasal bone
4 Parietal bone	12 Squamous part of temporal bone	19 Zygomatic bone
5 Parietal tuberosity		20 Greater wing of sphenoid
6 Lambdoid suture	13 Condylar process ⎤ of	21 Sphenoidal fontanelle
7 Occipital bone	14 Ramus ⎟ mandible	
8 Mastoid fontanelle	15 Body ⎦	

Normal postnatal closure of the six fontanelles:
➤ Sphenoidal (anterolateral) fontanelle (left and right) – 3 months
➤ Posterior (median) fontanelle – 3 months
➤ Mastoid (posterolateral) fontanelle (left and right) – 12 months
➤ Anterior (median) fontanelle – 18 months

Adult skull – *from the right*

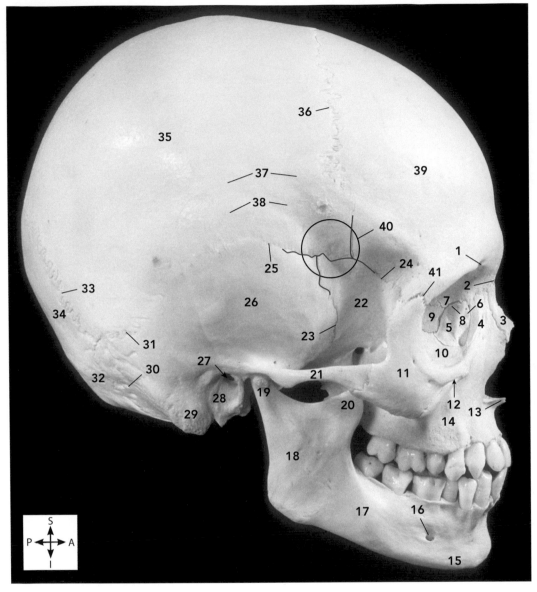

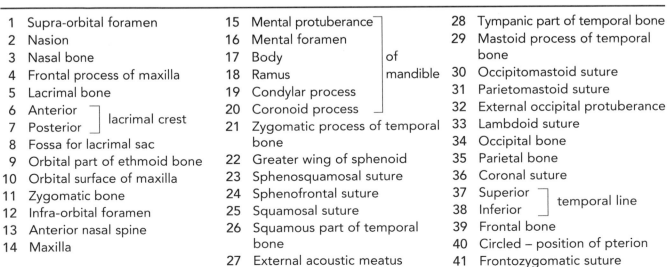

1	Supra-orbital foramen	15	Mental protuberance ⎤
2	Nasion	16	Mental foramen
3	Nasal bone	17	Body of
4	Frontal process of maxilla	18	Ramus mandible
5	Lacrimal bone	19	Condylar process
6	Anterior ⎤ lacrimal crest	20	Coronoid process ⎦
7	Posterior ⎦	21	Zygomatic process of temporal bone
8	Fossa for lacrimal sac	22	Greater wing of sphenoid
9	Orbital part of ethmoid bone	23	Sphenosquamosal suture
10	Orbital surface of maxilla	24	Sphenofrontal suture
11	Zygomatic bone	25	Squamosal suture
12	Infra-orbital foramen	26	Squamous part of temporal bone
13	Anterior nasal spine	27	External acoustic meatus
14	Maxilla		

28	Tympanic part of temporal bone
29	Mastoid process of temporal bone
30	Occipitomastoid suture
31	Parietomastoid suture
32	External occipital protuberance
33	Lambdoid suture
34	Occipital bone
35	Parietal bone
36	Coronal suture
37	Superior ⎤ temporal line
38	Inferior ⎦
39	Frontal bone
40	Circled – position of pterion
41	Frontozygomatic suture

Adult skull with individual bones coloured – *from the left*

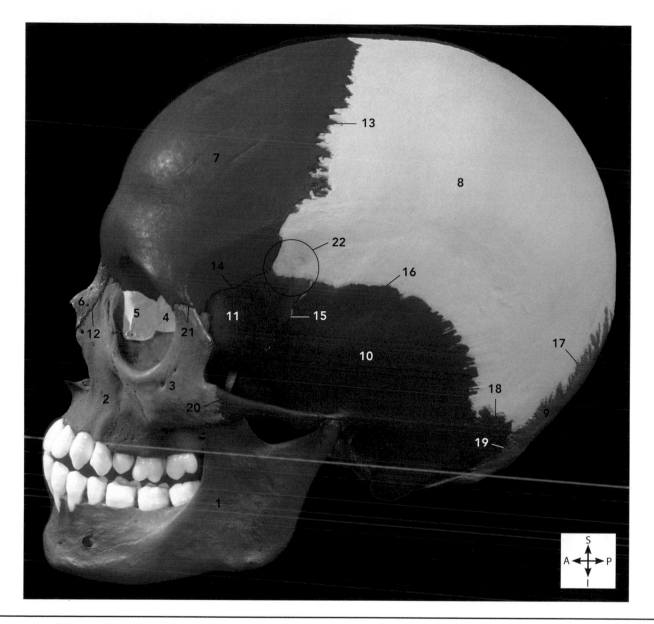

1	Mandible	9	Occipital bone
2	Maxilla	10	Temporal bone
3	Zygomatic bone	11	Sphenoid
4	Ethmoid bone	12	Nasomaxillary suture
5	Lacrimal bone	13	Coronal suture
6	Nasal bone	14	Sphenofrontal suture
7	Frontal bone	15	Sphenosquamosal suture
8	Parietal bone	16	Squamosal suture

17	Lambdoid suture
18	Parietomastoid suture
19	Occipitomastoid suture
20	Temporozygomatic suture
21	Frontozygomatic suture
22	Circled – position of pterion

Normal postnatal closure of the cranial sutures:
➤ Generally the sutures narrow by 6 months and then begin to interlock within the first year.
➤ They assume the adult typical serrated (meandering line) appearance by 2 years of age.
➤ Sutures fuse in the second decade and complete their ossification in the third decade.
➤ It is not uncommon for the two halves of the fetal frontal bone to fail to fuse resulting in a persistent frontal (metopic) suture.

Adult skull, median sagittal section hence removal of midline structures forming the nasal septum – *from the left*

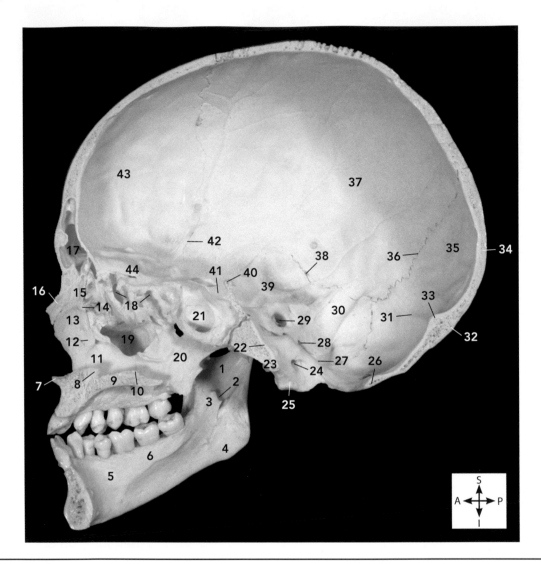

1 Ramus of mandible	18 Ethmoidal air cells	31 Groove for transverse sinus
2 Mandibular foramen	19 Maxillary sinus	32 External ⎤ occipital
3 Lingula ⎤	20 Medial pterygoid plate of sphenoid	33 Internal ⎦ protuberance
4 Angle ⎟	21 Sphenoidal sinus	34 Occiput
5 Body ⎬ of mandible	22 Clivus	35 Occipital bone
6 Mylohyoid line ⎦	23 Anterior margin of foramen magnum	36 Lambdoid suture
7 Anterior nasal spine of maxilla	24 Hypoglossal canal	37 Parietal bone
8 Nasal crest of maxilla	25 Mastoid process	38 Squamosal suture
9 Hard palate	26 Posterior margin of foramen magnum	39 Squamous part of temporal bone
10 Nasal crest of palatine bone	27 Jugular foramen	40 Dorsum sellae
11 Inferior meatus	28 Groove for inferior petrosal sinus	41 Sella turcica
12 Conchal crest	29 Internal acoustic meatus	42 Groove for middle meningeal vessels
13 Middle meatus	30 Groove for sigmoid sinus	43 Squamous ⎤ part of
14 Ethmoidal crest		44 Orbital ⎦ frontal bone
15 Frontal process of maxilla		
16 Nasal bone		
17 Frontal sinus		

Adult skull, median sagittal section with removal of the nasal septum and individual bones coloured – *from the right*

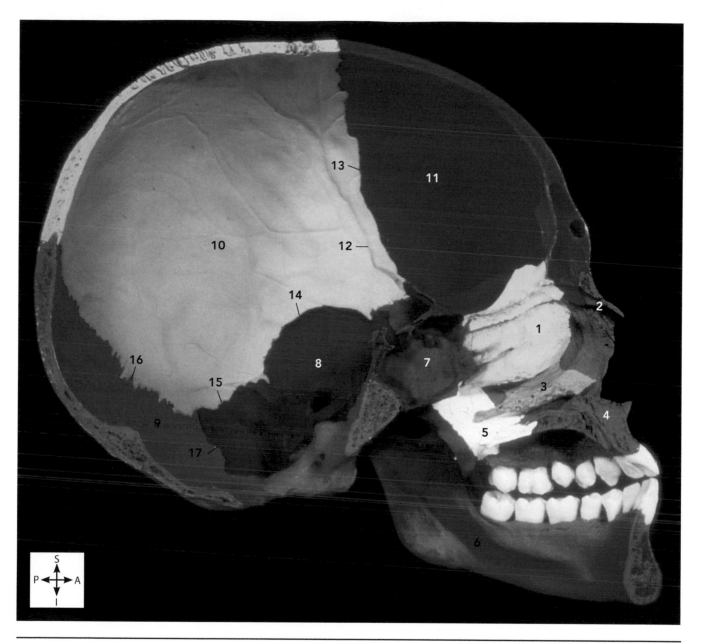

1	Ethmoid bone	8	Temporal bone	14	Squamosal suture
2	Nasal bone	9	Occipital bone	15	Parietomastoid suture
3	Inferior nasal concha	10	Parietal bone	16	Lambdoid suture
4	Maxilla	11	Frontal bone	17	Occipitomastoid suture
5	Palatine bone	12	Groove for middle meningeal		
6	Mandible		vessels		
7	Sphenoid	13	Coronal suture		

The nasal conchae:
➤ The superior and inferior nasal concha are integral parts of the ethmoid bone.
➤ The inferior nasal concha is an entirely separate bone that is attached by its anterior and posterior ends to the maxilla and palatine bone, respectively

Cranial vault coverings – *from above*

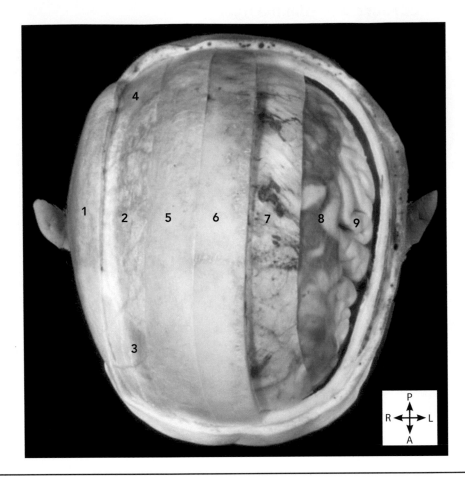

1 Skin and dense subcutaneous tissue
2 Epicranial aponeurosis
3 Frontal belly
4 Occipital belly ⎵ of occipitofrontalis
5 Loose connective tissue and pericranium

6 Bones of cranial vault
7 Dura mater
8 Arachnoid mater
9 Cerebral hemisphere covered by pia mater

The scalp consists of five distinct layers:
➤ Skin.
➤ Dense subcutaneous tissue.
➤ Epicranial aponeurosis and the two bellies of the occipitofrontalis muscle.
➤ Loose connective tissue.
➤ Pericranium (periosteum of cranial vault).

The cranial vault:
➤ Is formed by the union of the frontal, occipital and two parietal bones.

The meninges:
➤ Comprise the three connective tissue membranes that line both the cranial cavity and vertebral canal to enclose both the brain and spinal cord.
➤ The *dura mater* is the outermost and by far the thickest of the meninges. It has a *cerebral* part that lines the cranium and has an outer endosteal layer and an inner meningeal layer; although the two layers adhere tightly together with one another, in certain areas they separate to form distinct cavities, the venous sinuses; and a *spinal part*, continuous with the cerebral part, forms a tubular sheath within the length of the vertebral column.
➤ The *arachnoid mater* lies inside the dura mater, separated from it by the subdural space.
➤ The *pia mater* is the thinnest of all the membranes and it adheres tightly to the surface of both the brain and spinal cord.

Brain, with arachnoid mater and underlying blood vessels removed from the right hemisphere – *from above*

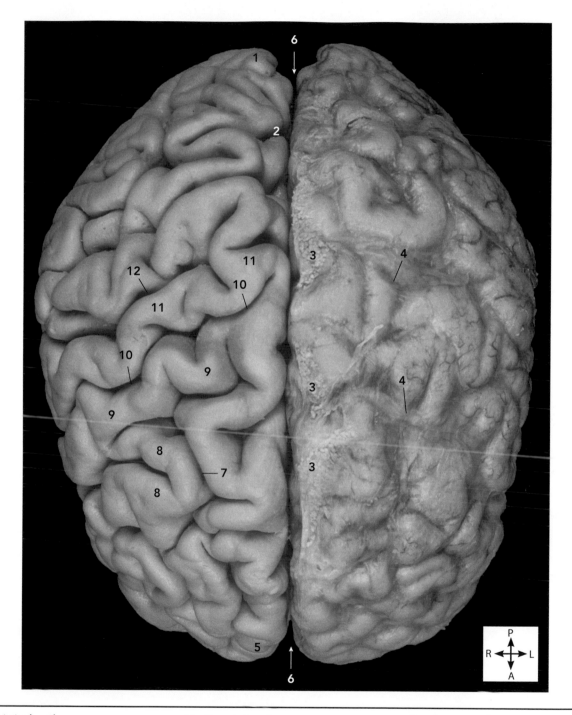

1	Occipital pole	5	Frontal pole
2	Parieto-occipital sulcus	6	Longitudinal cerebral fissure
3	Arachnoid granulations	7	Superior frontal sulcus
4	Superior cerebral veins	8	Middle frontal gyrus

9	Precentral gyrus
10	Central sulcus
11	Postcentral gyrus
12	Postcentral sulcus

The cerebral cortex:
➤ Is formed into smooth, broad, convoluted folds that are termed gyri (singular gyrus).
➤ The spaces between the gyri are termed sulci (singular sulcus).

Brain, with arachnoid mater covering intact – *from the left*

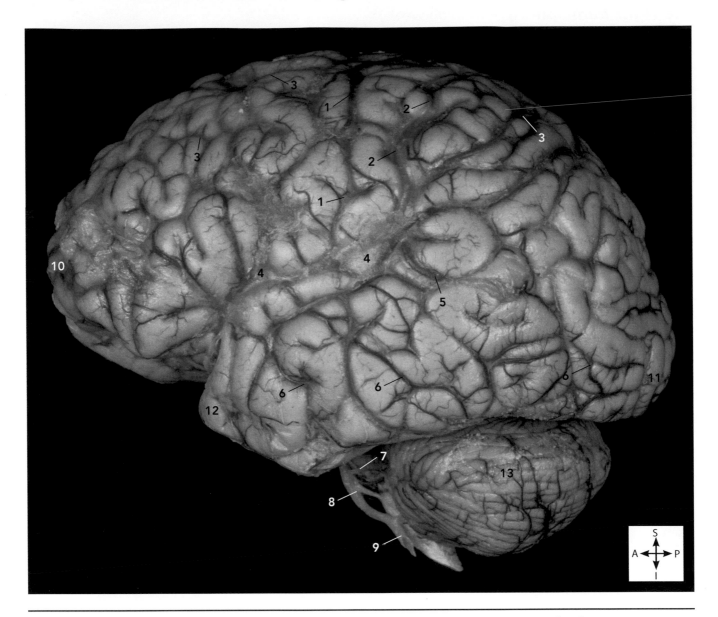

1 Artery of central sulcus	6 Inferior cerebral veins	11 Occipital pole
2 Superior anastomotic vein	7 Superior cerebral artery	12 Temporal pole
3 Superior cerebral veins	8 Basilar artery	13 Cerebral hemisphere
4 Lateral sulcus	9 Vertebral artery	
5 Inferior anastomotic vein	10 Frontal pole	

The cerebellar cortex:
➤ Consists of multiple folds, much finer in structure than that of the cerebrum, termed *folia* and are not individually named.

Brain, with arachnoid mater and underlying blood vessels removed –

from the left

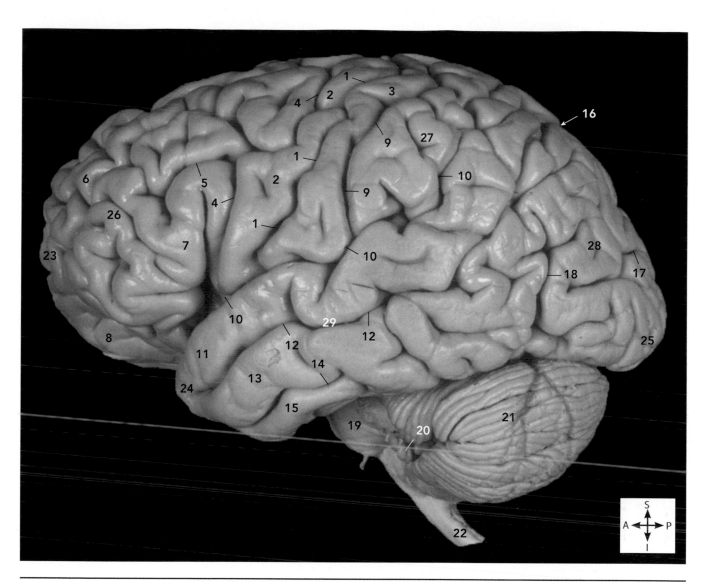

1	Central sulcus	11	Superior temporal gyrus	21	Cerebellar hemisphere
2	Precentral gyrus	12	Superior temporal sulcus	22	Medulla oblongata
3	Postcentral gyrus	13	Middle temporal gyrus	23	Frontal pole
4	Precentral sulcus	14	Inferior temporal sulcus	24	Temporal pole
5	Inferior frontal sulcus	15	Inferior temporal gyrus	25	Occipital pole
6	Superior frontal sulcus	16	Parieto-occipital sulcus	26	Frontal lobe
7	Inferior frontal gyrus	17	Lunate sulcus	27	Parietal lobe
8	Orbital gyri	18	Anterior occipital sulcus	28	Occipital lobe
9	Postcentral sulcus	19	Pons	29	Temporal lobe
10	Lateral sulcus	20	Flocculus		

Brain, median sagittal section, with arachnoid covering intact – *from the right*

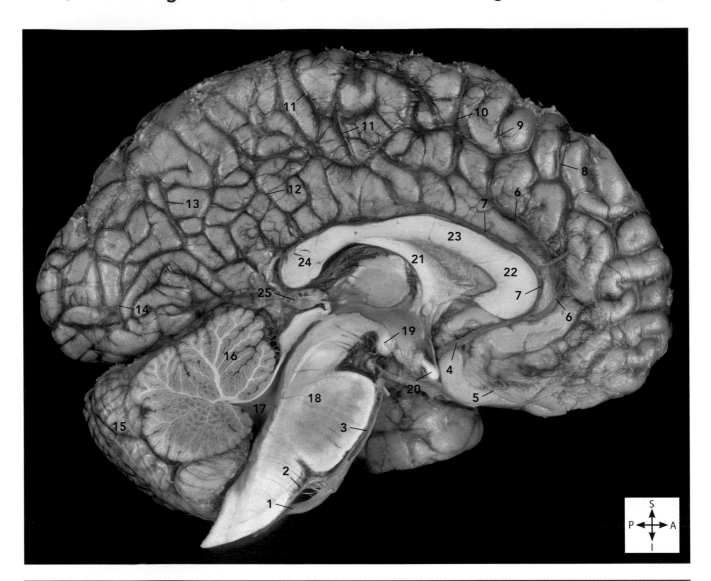

1	Left vertebral artery	9	Intermediomedial frontal artery	17	Fourth ventricle
2	Anterior inferior cerebellar artery	10	Posteromedial frontal artery	18	Pons
3	Basilar artery	11	Paracentral artery	19	Mamillary body
4	Anterior cerebellar artery	12	Precuneal artery	20	Optic nerve (II)
5	Medial frontobasal artery	13	Parieto-occipital branch ⎤ of posterior	21	Body of fornix
6	Callosomarginal artery		⎥ cerebral	22	Genu ⎤ of corpus
7	Pericallosal artery	14	Calcarine branch ⎦ artery	23	Body ⎥ callosum
8	Anteromedial frontal artery	15	Cerebellar hemisphere	24	Splenium ⎦
		16	Anterior lobe of cerebellum	25	Pineal body

The brain consists of the:
➤ Cerebrum.
➤ Brainstem.
➤ Cerebellum.

The cerebrum has two cerebral hemispheres each with a:
➤ Frontal, parietal, occipital, temporal, insula (insular lobe) and limbic lobe.

The brainstem consists of:
➤ Midbrain.
➤ Pons.
➤ Medulla oblongata.

The midbrain consists of:
➤ The two cerebral peduncles.

Brain, median sagittal section, with arachnoid and underlying blood vessels removed – *from the right*

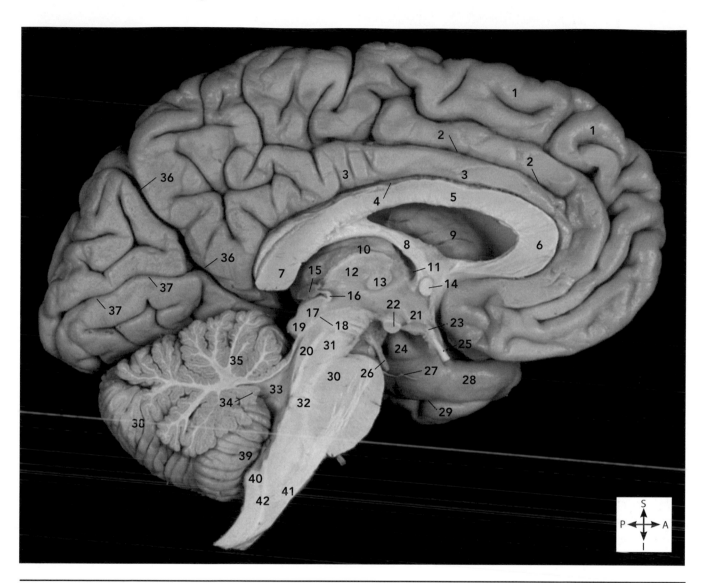

1	Superior frontal gyrus	14	Anterior commisure	30	Pons
2	Cingulate sulcus	15	Pineal body	31	Midbrain
3	Cingulate gyrus	16	Posterior commisure	32	Pontine tegmentum
4	Corpus callosal sulcus	17	Superior calliculus	33	Fourth ventricle
5	Body ⎤ of corpus	18	Aqueduct of midbrain	34	Nodulus
6	Genu ⎥ callosum	19	Inferior calliculus	35	Anterior lobe of cerebellum
7	Splenium ⎦	20	Mesencephalon	36	Parieto-occipital fissure
8	Body of fornix	21	Hypothalamus	37	Calcarine sulcus
9	Caudate nucleus (head) in wall of lateral ventricle	22	Mamillary body	38	Cerebellar hemisphere
		23	Infundibulum	39	Tonsil of cerebellum
10	Third ventricle	24	Uncus	40	Inferior cerebellar peduncle
11	Foramen of habenular commisure	25	Optic nerve (II)	41	Pyramid of medulla oblongata
		26	Oculomotor nerve (III)		
12	Thalamus	27	Trochlear nerve (IV)	42	Medulla oblongata
13	Massa intermedia (interthalmic adhesion)	28	Parahippocampal gyrus		
		29	Rhinal sulcus		

Dura mater and meningeal vessels – *from the left*

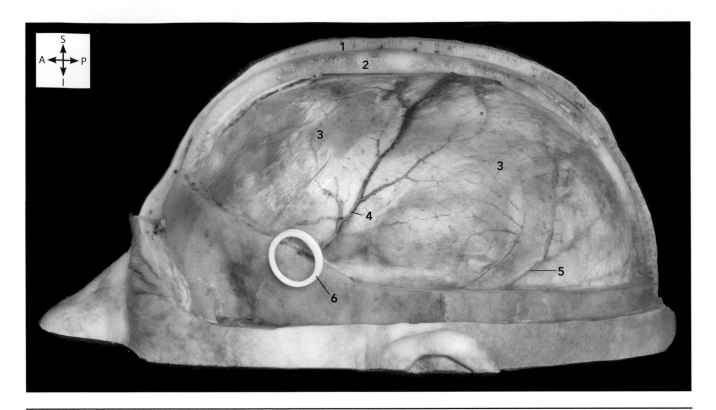

1	Skin and dense subcutaneous tissue of scalp	4	Anterior branch ⎤
2	Bones of cranial vault	5	Posterior branch ⎦ of middle meningeal artery
3	Dura mater	6	Position of pterion (circled)

The pterion:
➤ Is an area identifiable by a distinct 'H'-shaped arrangement of cranial bone sutures formed by the union of the frontal bone, parietal bone, squamous part of the temporal bone and greater wing of the sphenoid.
➤ It is a very important landmark because it immediately overlies the anterior branch of the middle meningeal artery, a vessel prone to severe damage (rupture) by a blow to the side of the head.

Cranial cavity, paramedian sagittal section, hence the preservation of the falx cerebri and nasal septum – *from the right*

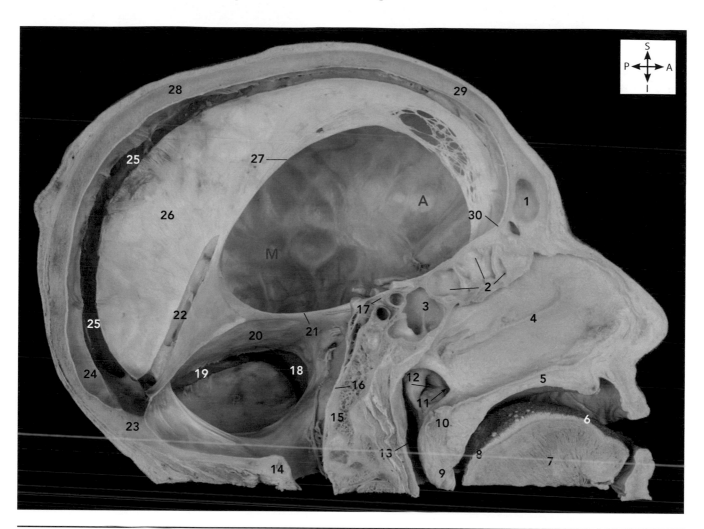

A	Anterior ⎤	9	Uvula
M	Middle ⎬ cranial fossa	10	Soft palate
P	Posterior ⎦	11	Posterior nasal aperture
		12	Opening of auditory tube
1	Frontal sinus	13	Nasal part of pharynx (nasopharynx)
2	Ethmoidal air cells	14	Posterior ⎤ of foramen
3	Sphenoidal sinus	15	Anterior margin ⎦ magnum
4	Nasal septum	16	Clivus
5	Hard palate	17	Pituitary gland
6	Presulcal part of dorsum of tongue	18	Sigmoid sinus
7	Genioglossus	19	Transverse sinus
8	Postsulcal part of dorsum of tongue	20	Tentorium cerebelli

21	Free margin of tentorium cerebelli
22	Straight sinus
23	Internal occipital protuberance
24	Occipital bone
25	Superior sagittal sinus
26	Falx cerebri
27	Inferior margin of falx cerebri
28	Parietal bone
29	Frontal bone
30	Crista galli of ethmoid bone

Base of adult skull, external surface – *from below*

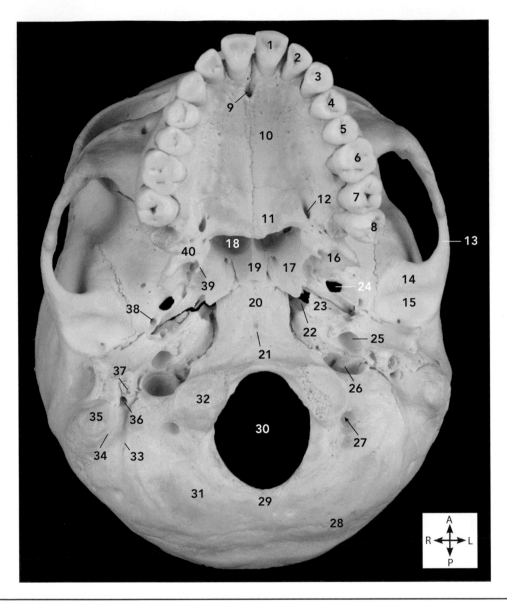

1	First central incisor	16	Lateral ⎤ pterygoid plate	31	Occipital bone
2	Second lateral incisor	17	Medial ⎦	32	Occipital condyle
3	Canine	18	Posterior nasal aperture	33	Occipital groove
4	First ⎤ premolar	19	Vomer	34	Mastoid notch
5	Second ⎦	20	Body of sphenoid	35	Mastoid process
6	First ⎤ molar	21	Pharyngeal tubercle	36	Stylomastoid foramen
7	Second ⎥	22	Foramen lacerum	37	Styloid process
8	Third ⎦	23	Apex of petrous part of temporal bone	38	Foramen spinosum
9	Incisive fossa	24	Foramen ovale	39	Pterygoid hamulus
10	Palatine process of maxilla	25	Carotid canal	40	Pyramidal process of palatine bone
11	Horizontal plate of palatine bone	26	Jugular foramen		
12	Greater palatine foramina	27	Condylar canal		
13	Zygomatic process ⎤ of temporal bone	28	Superior nuchal line		
14	Articular tubercle ⎥	29	External occipital crest		
15	Mandibular fossa ⎦	30	Foramen magnum		

Base of adult skull, internal surface – *from above*

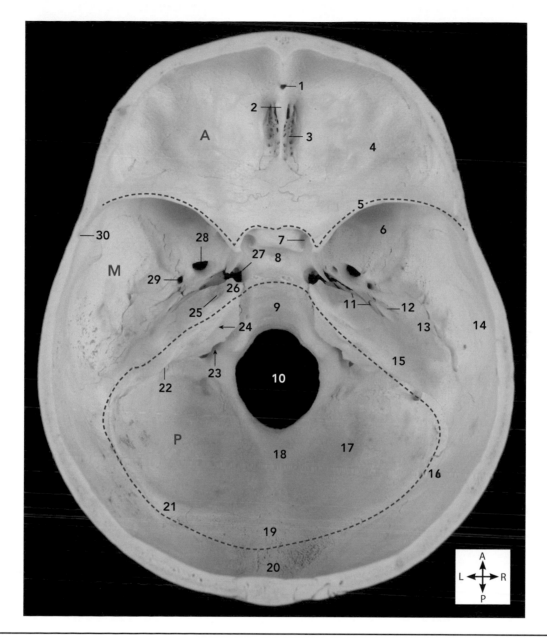

A Anterior	11 Hiatus and groove for greater petrosal nerve	21 Groove for transverse sinus
M Middle } cranial fossa	12 Hiatus and groove for lesser petrosal nerve	22 Groove for sigmoid sinus
P Posterior	13 Tegmen tympani	23 Jugular foramen
	14 Squamous } of temporal bone	24 Internal acoustic meatus
1 Foramen caecum	15 Petrous part } bone	25 Trigeminal impression
2 Crista galli } of ethmoid	16 Mastoid angle of parietal bone	26 Apex of petrous part of temporal bone
3 Cribriform plate } bone	17 Occipital bone	27 Foramen lacerum
4 Orbital part of frontal bone	18 Internal occipital crest	28 Foramen ovale
5 Lesser } wing	19 Internal occipital protuberance	29 Foramen spinosum
6 Greater } of sphenoid	20 Groove for superior sagittal sinus	30 Groove for frontal branch of middle meningeal artery and vein
7 Optic canal		
8 Sella turcica		
9 Clivus		
10 Foramen magnum		

Brain, base, cerebellum and brainstem, with arachnoid mater and blood vessels removed from the left hemisphere – *from below*

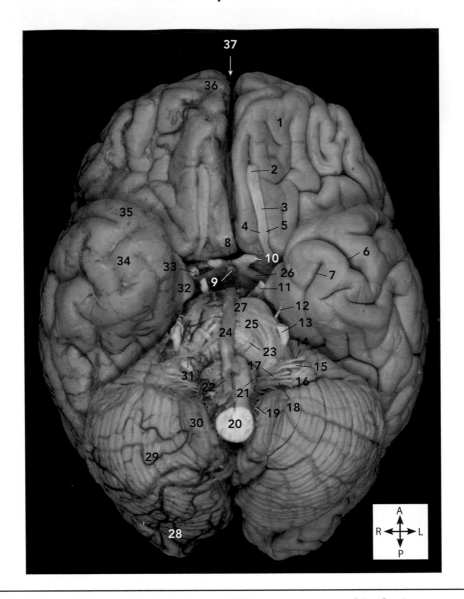

1 Inferior surface of frontal lobe	14 Facial nerve (VII)	26 Optic tract
2 Olfactory bulb	15 Vestibulocochlear nerve (VII)	27 Mamillary body
3 Olfactory tract	16 Flocculus	28 Occipital pole
4 Medial ⎤ olfactory stria	17 Glossopharyngeal nerve (IX)	29 Cerebellum
5 Lateral ⎦	18 Vagus nerve (X)	30 Tonsil of cerebellum
6 Inferior temporal sulcus	19 Cranial part of accessory nerve (XI)	31 Labyrinthine artery
7 Collateral sulcus	20 Medulla oblongata	32 Parahippocampal gyrus
8 Optic chiasma	21 Hypoglossal nerve (XII)	33 Internal carotid artery
9 Infundibulum	22 Vertebral artery	34 Inferior surface of temporal pole
10 Optic nerve (II)	23 Abducent nerve (VI)	35 Temporal pole
11 Oculomotor nerve (III)	24 Basilar artery	36 Frontal pole
12 Trochlear nerve (IV)	25 Pons	37 Longitudinal cerebral fissure
13 Trigeminal nerve (V)		

A Cranial cavity, base – *from above*

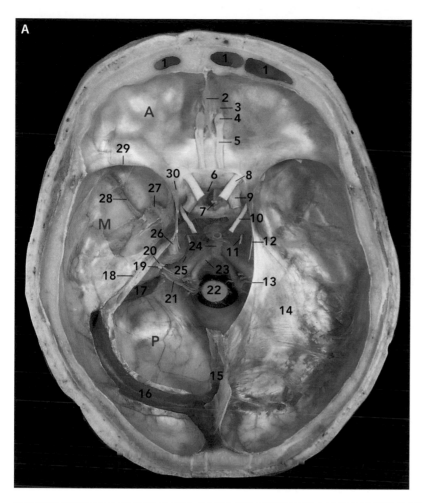

B Isolated pituitary gland, actual size as presented at dissection

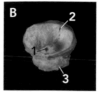

1 Infundibulum of pituitary stalk
2 Adenohypophysis (anterior) ⎤ lobe of
3 Neurohypophysis (posterior) ⎦ pituitary gland

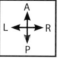

For images A, B

A Anterior ⎤	
M Middle ⎬ cranial fossa	
P Posterior ⎦	

1 Frontal sinus
2 Crista galli of ethmoid bone
3 Olfactory nerve filaments (I)
4 Olfactory bulb
5 Olfactory tract
6 Diaphragma sellae
7 Infundibulum
8 Optic nerve (II)
9 Internal carotid artery
10 Oculomotor nerve (III)

11 Abducent nerve (VI)
12 Trochlear nerve (IV)
13 Free margin of tentorium cerebelli
14 Tentorium cerebelli
15 Straight sinus at junction of falx cerebri and tentorium cerebelli
16 Transverse sinus
17 Sigmoid sinus
18 Superior petrosal sinus and cut edges of attached margins of tentorium cerebelli
19 Vestibulocochlear nerve (VIII)
20 Facial nerve (VII)

21 Spinal root of accessory nerve (XI)
22 Medulla oblongata
23 Vertebral artery
24 Basilar artery
25 Inferior petrosal sinus
26 Trigeminal nerve (V)
27 Mandibular nerve (V3)
28 Middle meningeal artery
29 Posterior margin of lesser wing of sphenoid
30 Anterior clinoid process

Main blood supply to the brain is via:
➤ The *vertebral arteries.*
➤ The *internal carotid arteries.*
➤ A series of communicating vessels between the vertebral and internal carotid arteries form a ring-like anastomosis on the undersurface of the brain to create the arterial *circle of Willis.*

Cranial cavity, brain and upper spinal cord in a paramedian sagittal section, with removal of the falx cerebri and nasal septum – *from the right*

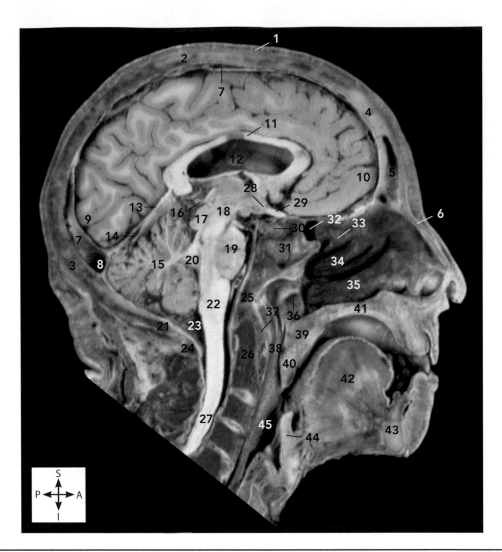

1	Skin and dense subcutaneous tissue of scalp	
2	Parietal bone	
3	Occipital bone	
4	Frontal bone	
5	Frontal sinus	
6	Nasal bone	
7	Superior sagittal sinus	
8	Transverse sinus	
9	Occipital ⎤ pole	
10	Frontal ⎦	
11	Corpus callosum	
12	Lateral ventricle	
13	Tentorium cerebelli	
14	Straight sinus	
15	Cerebellar hemisphere	
16	Pineal body	
17	Midbrain	
18	Brainstem	
19	Pons	
20	Fourth ventricle	
21	Posterior margin of foramen magnum	
22	Medulla oblongata	
23	Cisterna magna	
24	Posterior arch of atlas (first [CI] cervical vertebra)	
25	Anterior margin of foramen magnum	
26	Dens of axis (second [CII] cervical vertebra)	
27	Spinal medulla (spinal cord)	
28	Optic chiasma	
29	Optic nerve (II)	
30	Pituitary gland	
31	Sphenoidal sinus	
32	Spheno-ethmoidal recess	
33	Superior ⎤	
34	Middle ⎬ nasal concha	
35	Inferior ⎦	
36	Opening of auditory tube	
37	Anterior arch of atlas (first [CI] cervical vertebra)	
38	Nasal part of pharynx (nasopharynx)	
39	Soft palate	
40	Uvula	
41	Hard palate	
42	Genioglossus	
43	Body of mandible	
44	Epiglottis	
45	Oral part of pharynx (oropharynx)	

Cranial cavity, brain and upper spinal cord in a paramedian sagittal section, with removal of the falx cerebri and nasal septum and exposure of cranial nerves *in situ* – *from the right*

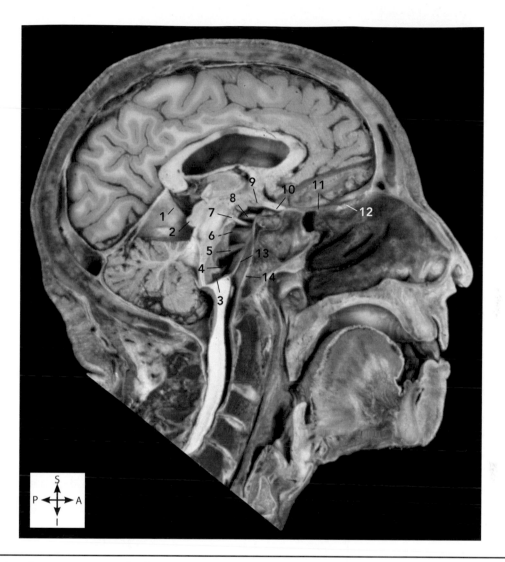

1 Free margin of tentorium cerebelli	7 Oculomotor nerve (III)
2 Inferior colliculus	8 Ophthalmic artery
3 Glossopharyngeal nerve (IX), vagus nerve (X), cranial part of accessory nerve (XI)	9 Optic chiasma
	10 Optic nerve (II)
4 Facial nerve (VII), vestibulocochlear nerve (VIII)	11 Olfactory tract
5 Trigeminal nerve (V)	12 Olfactory bulb
6 Trochlear nerve (IV) on free margin of tentorium cerebelli	13 Abducent nerve (VI)
	14 Clivus

Cranial cavity, cavernous sinus, cranial nerves *in situ* – *from the left above and slightly behind*

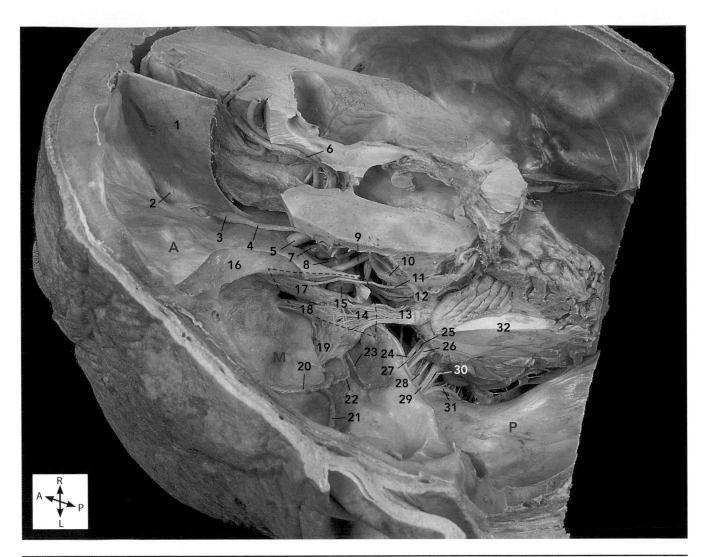

A	Anterior ⎤	
M	Middle	cranial fossa
P	Posterior ⎦	

Dotted area denotes extent of the cavernous sinus

1 Falx cerebri
2 Falx cerebri attached to crista galli of ethmoid bone
3 Olfactory bulb
4 Olfactory tract
5 Optic nerve (II)
6 Cortical branches of middle cerebral artery

7 Ophthalmic artery
8 Pituitary gland
9 Oculomotor nerve (III)
10 Posterior cerebellar artery
11 Trochlear nerve (IV)
12 Superior cerebellar artery
13 Trigeminal nerve (V)
14 Trigeminal ganglion
15 Internal carotid artery
16 Posterior margin of lesser wing of sphenoid bone
17 Ophthalmic nerve (V¹)
18 Maxillary nerve (V²)
19 Mandibular nerve (V³)

20 Frontal ⎤ branch of middle
21 Parietal ⎦ meningeal artery
22 Lesser ⎤ petrosal nerve
23 Greater ⎦
24 Facial nerve (VII)
25 Labyrinthine artery
26 Vestibulocochlear nerve (VIII)
27 Nervous intermedius
28 Glossopharyngeal nerve (IX)
29 Vagus nerve (X)
30 Cranial part ⎤ of accessory
31 Spinal root ⎦ nerve (XI)
32 Cerebellar hemisphere

Cranial cavity, optic and olfactory nerves *in situ* – *from above*

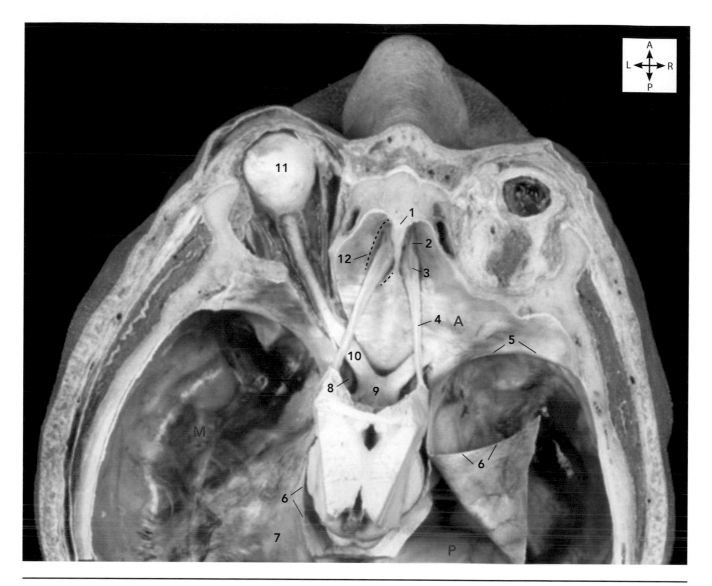

A	Anterior		4	Olfactory tract	8	Ophthalmic artery
M	Middle	cranial fossa	5	Posterior margin of lesser wing of sphenoid	9	Optic chiasma
P	Posterior				10	Optic nerve (II)
			6	Free margin of tentorium cerebelli (reflected superiorly on right side)	11	Eyeball within orbital cavity
1	Crista galli of ethmoid bone				12	Cribriform plate of ethmoid bone (outlined)
2	Filaments of olfactory nerves (I)					
3	Olfactory bulb		7	Tentorium cerebelli		

Olfactory nerve (I):

➤ Not a single nerve as the name implies, but numerous fine nerve filaments enseathed in dura that pass through the roof of the nose into the anterior cranial fossa via multiple foramina within the cribriform plate of the ethmoid bone.

➤ The nerve filaments then enter the under-surface of the olfactory bulb.

Lower brainstem and cervical part of the spinal cord – *from behind*

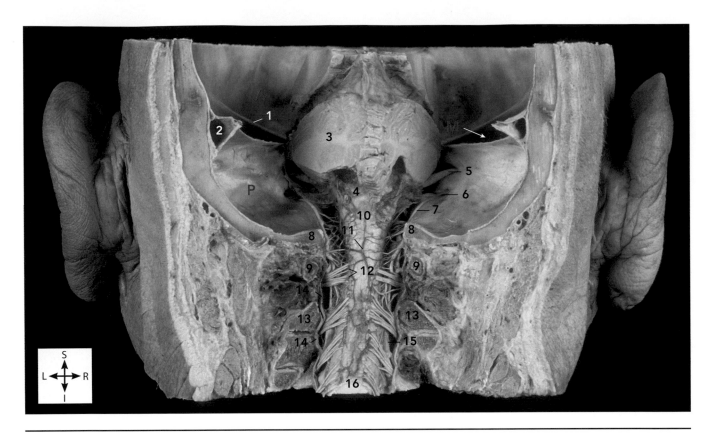

A Anterior ⎤	6 Glossopharyngeal nerve (IX), vagus nerve (X), accessory nerves (XI), in jugular foramen	11 Posterior spinal arteries within arachnoid mater
M Middle ⎬ cranial fossa	7 Spinal root of accessory nerve (XI)	12 Dorsal rootlets of second cervical nerve
P Posterior ⎦	8 Margin of foramen magnum	13 Lamina of axis (second [CII] cervical vertebra)
1 Posterior margin of lesser wing of sphenoid	9 Posterior arch of atlas (first [CI] cervical vertebra)	14 Dura mater (cut edge)
2 Transverse sinus	10 Medulla oblongata	15 Ligamentum denticulatum
3 Cerebellum		16 Spinal medulla (spinal cord)
4 Tela choroidea and choroid plexus		
5 Facial nerve (VII), vestibulocochlear nerve (VIII) and labyrinthine artery, in internal acoustic meatus		

The medulla oblongata:
➤ Passes through the foramen magnum to become continuous with the spinal medulla (spinal cord).

Lower brainstem and cervical part of the spinal cord – *from behind*

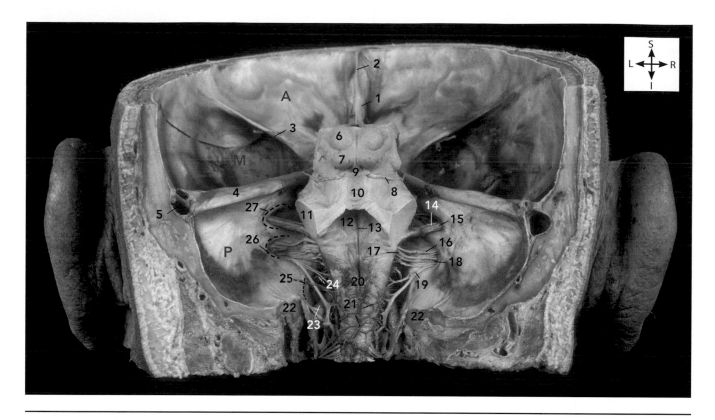

A	Anterior	8	Trochlear nerve (IV)
M	Middle — cranial fossa	9	Superior medullary vellum
P	Posterior	10	Lingula

		11	Cerebellar peduncle
1	Crista galli of ethmoid bone	12	Floor of fourth ventricle
2	Falx cerebri	13	Median groove
3	Posterior margin of lesser wing of sphenoid	14	Facial nerve (VII)
4	Tentorium cerebelli (reflected anteriorly)	15	Vestibulocochlear nerve (VIII)
5	Transverse sinus	16	Glossopharyngeal nerve (IX)
6	Superior — colliculus	17	Vagus nerve (X)
7	Inferior	18	Cranial part of accessory nerve (XI)

19	Spinal root of accessory nerve (XI)
20	Medulla oblongata
21	Posterior spinal arteries within arachnoid mater
22	Margin of foramen magnum
23	Vertebral artery
24	Hypoglossal nerve (XII)
25	Hypoglossal canal
26	Jugular foramen
27	Internal acoustic meatus

A Superficial structures of the head, neck, shoulder and upper thorax –
from the front and left

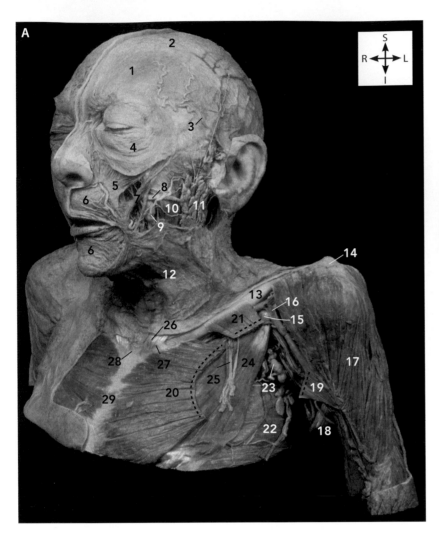

B An isolated cluster of lateral axillary lymph nodes with associated vessels, actual size as presented at dissection

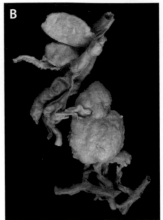

1 Frontal belly of occipitofrontalis	13 Clavicle (body)	22 Serratus anterior
2 Epicranial aponeurosis	14 Position of acromioclavicular joint	23 Axillary lymph nodes (cluster)
3 Superficial temporal artery	15 Position of coracoid process of scapula	24 Pectoralis minor
4 Orbicularis oculi		25 Thoraco-acromial vessels and lateral pectoral nerve
5 Zygomaticus major	16 Cephalic vein in deltopectoral triangle	26 Sternocleidomastoid (sternal head)
6 Orbicularis oris	17 Deltoid	27 Position of sternoclavicular joint
7 Zygomaticus minor	18 Latissimus dorsi	
8 Parotid duct	19 Pectoralis major (common origin)	28 Suprasternal notch
9 Buccal fat pad	20 Sternocostal ⎤ part of	29 Body of sternum
10 Masseter	21 Clavicular ⎦ pectoralis major	
11 Parotid gland		
12 Platysma		

Lymph nodes:
➤ Are sited regionally throughout the body and may be found as singleton, pairs or in distinct multiple cluster groups.
➤ Nodes are usually small, ovoid or kidney (reniform) in shape and vary between 0.1 and 2.5 cm in length.
➤ Some nodes, but not all, may be palpable in their normal state, but particularly so when diseased.

Anterior cervical region (anterior triangle) of neck – *from the front and left*

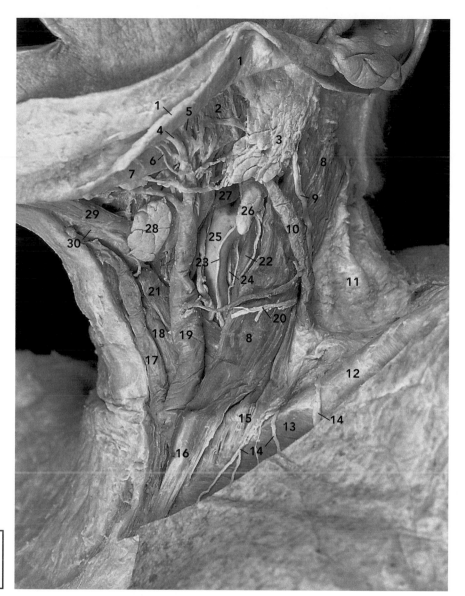

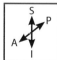

1	Platysma (reflected superiorly)	
2	Masseter	
3	Parotid gland	
4	Facial artery	
5	Facial vein	
6	Marginal mandibular branch of the facial nerve	
7	Body of mandible	
8	Sternocleidomastoid	
9	Great auricular nerve	
10	External jugular vein	

11	Prevertebral fascia overlying levator scapulae
12	Clavicle (body)
13	Clavicular part of pectoralis major
14	Supraclavicular nerves
15	Clavicular head ⎤ of
16	Sternal head ⎦ sternocleidomastoid
17	Anterior jugular vein
18	Sternothyroid
19	Internal jugular vein
20	Transverse cervical nerve
21	Omohyoid

22	Internal jugular vein
23	Superior root of ansa cervicalis
24	Vagus nerve
25	Common carotid artery
26	Jugulodigastric lymph node
27	Posterior belly of digastric
28	Submandibular gland (unusually low)
29	Anterior belly of digastric
30	Mylohyoid

Boundaries of the anterior cervical region (anterior triangle) of neck are:
➤ The anterior border of the sternocleidomastoid, the lower border of the mandible and the midline.

Lateral cervical region (posterior triangle) of neck – *from the front, left and above*

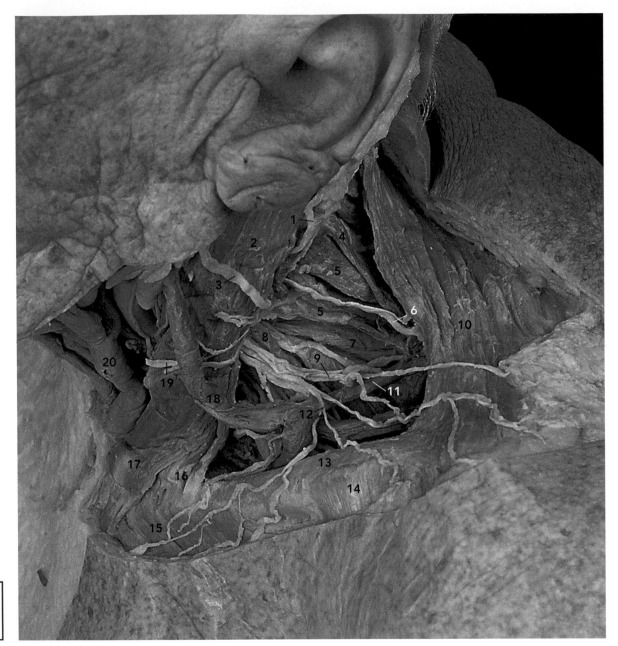

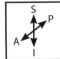

1 Lesser occipital nerve	9 Cervical nerves to trapezius	15 Sternocostal part of pectoralis major
2 Sternocleidomastoid	10 Trapezius	16 Clavicular ⎤ head of
3 Greater auricular nerve	11 Superficial cervical vein	17 Sternal ⎦ sternocleidomastoid
4 Splenius capitis	12 Supraclavicular nerves	18 External jugular vein
5 Levator scapulae	13 Clavicle (body)	19 Transverse cervical nerve
6 Accessory nerve	14 Clavicular part of pectoralis major	20 Anterior jugular vein
7 Posterior ⎤ scalene		
8 Middle ⎦		

Boundaries of the lateral cervical region (posterior triangle) of the neck are:
➤ The posterior border of the sternocleidomastoid, the anterior border of the trapezius and the middle third of the clavicle.

A Deep neck, great vessels – *from the front*

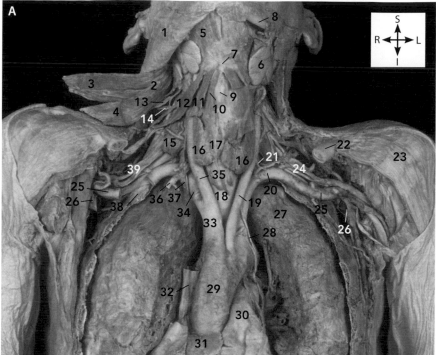

B Isolated thyroid gland, actual size as presented at dissection – *from above*

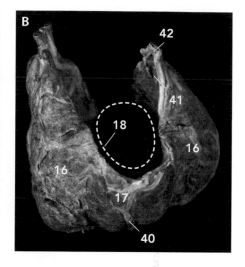

C Isolated left superior parathyroid gland, actual size as presented at dissection – *from the right*

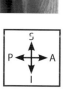

1 Platysma (reflected supero-laterally)	17 Isthmus of thyroid gland	32 Superior vena cava
2 Sternocleidomastoid (reflected laterally)	18 Trachea	33 Brachiocephalic artery
3 Sternal ⎤ head of sternocleidomastoid	19 Left common carotid artery	34 Right subclavian artery
4 Clavicular ⎦ (reflected laterally)	20 Left subclavian artery	35 Right common carotid artery
5 Anterior belly of digastric	21 Inferior thyroid artery	36 Internal thoracic artery
6 Submandibular gland	22 Clavicle (body)	37 Phrenic nerve
7 Body of hyoid bone	23 Deltoid	38 First (I) rib
8 Body of mandible	24 Left brachial plexus	39 Right brachial plexus
9 Laryngeal prominence of thyroid cartilage	25 Axillary artery	40 Inferior thyroid vein
10 Sternohyoid	26 Axillary vein	41 Left superior parathyroid gland
11 Sternothyroid	27 Apex of lung	42 Left superior thyroid artery and vein
12 Superior belly of omohyoid	28 Vagus nerve	
13 Great auricular nerve	29 Ascending aorta	
14 Accessory nerve	30 Pulmonary trunk	
15 Scalenus anterior	31 Auricle of right atrium	
16 Lateral lobe of thyroid gland		

A Deep structures of neck I – *from the left and slightly below*

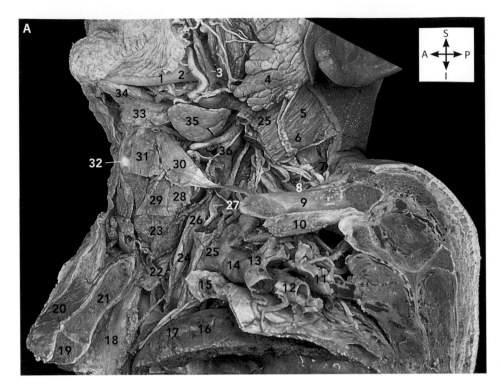

B Isolated left submandibular gland, actual size as presented at dissection – *from above*

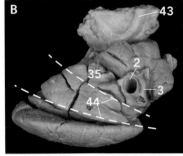

C Isolated left parotid gland, actual size as presented at dissection – *from above*

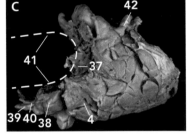

For images B, C

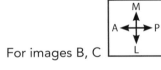

1 Body of mandible	16 Apex of lung	30 Superior belly of omohyoid
2 Facial artery	17 Internal thoracic artery and vein	31 Sternohyoid
3 Facial vein	18 Residual thymus	32 Laryngeal prominence of thyroid cartilage
4 Parotid gland (superficial part)	19 Body of sternum	33 Body of hyoid bone
5 Sternocleidomastoid	20 Sternal angle and manubriosternal joint	34 Anterior belly of digastric
6 Great auricular nerve	21 Manubrium of sternum	35 Submandibular gland
7 Accessory nerve	22 Inferior thyroid vein	36 Superior thyroid artery and vein
8 Cervical nerve branches to trapezius	23 Lateral lobe of thyroid gland	37 Maxillary artery
9 Clavicle (body)	24 Common carotid artery	38 Accessory parotid gland
10 Subclavius	25 Internal jugular vein	39 Parotid duct
11 Brachial plexus	26 Superior thyroid artery and vein	40 Buccal branch of facial nerve
12 Subclavian artery	27 Vagus nerve	41 Position of ramus of mandible
13 Suprascapular and transverse cervical veins	28 Sternothyroid	42 Parotid gland (deep part)
14 Subclavian vein	29 Thyrohyoid	43 Submandibular duct
15 First (I) rib		44 Position of body of mandible

Deep structures of neck II, with bisection and removal of the left half of pharynx and larynx – *from the front left and slightly below*

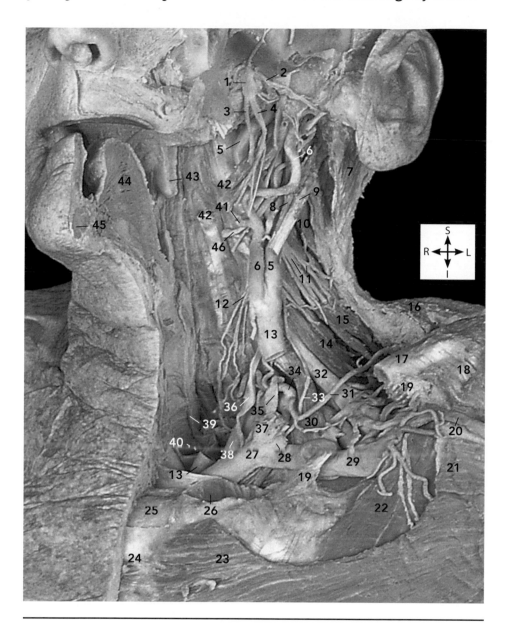

10 Splenius capitis
11 Cervical nerve ventral rami
12 Sympathetic trunk
13 Common carotid artery
14 Middle scalene
15 Levator scapulae
16 Trapezius
17 Clavicle (body)
18 Deltoid
19 Subclavius
20 Cephalic vein within deltopectoral triangle
21 Clavicular head of pectoralis major
22 Pectoralis minor
23 Sternal head of pectoralis major
24 Manubrium of sternum
25 Suprasternal notch
26 Disc of sternoclavicular joint
27 Brachiocephalic vein
28 Thoracic duct
29 Subclavian vein
30 Anterior scalene
31 Transverse cervical artery
32 Upper trunk of brachial plexus
33 Phrenic nerve
34 Thyrocervical trunk
35 Stellate ganglion
36 Vagus nerve
37 Internal jugular vein
38 Subclavian artery
39 Oesophagus
40 Trachea
41 Facial artery
42 Longus capitis
43 Uvula
44 Genioglossus
45 Body of mandible
46 Hypoglossal nerve

1 Mandibular nerve (V³)
2 Auriculotemporal nerve
3 Lingual nerve
4 Inferior alveolar nerve
5 Internal ⎤
6 External ⎦ carotid artery
7 Sternocleidomastoid
8 Stylohyoid
9 Posterior belly of digastric

Face, superficial structures I – *from the left*

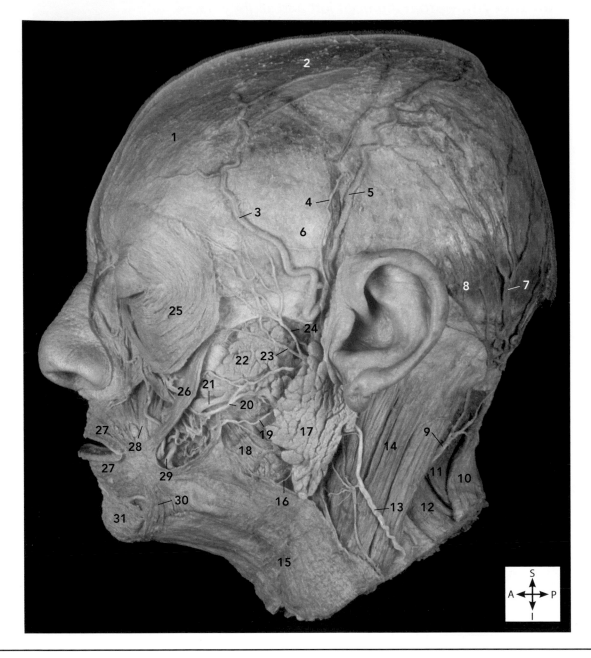

1 Frontal belly of occipitofrontalis	9 Lesser occipital nerve	21 Parotid duct
2 Epicranial aponeurosis	10 Trapezius	22 Accessory parotid gland
3 Frontal branch of superficial temporal artery	11 Splenius capitis	23 Zygomatic branch of facial nerve
4 Auriculotemporal nerve	12 Levator scapulae	24 Temporal branch of facial nerve
5 Parietal branch of superficial temporal artery	13 Great auricular nerve	
6 Temporal fascia overlying temporalis	14 Sternocleidomastoid	25 Orbicularis oculi
7 Occipital artery	15 Platysma	26 Zygomaticus major
	16 Cervical branch of facial nerve	27 Orbicularis oris
8 Occipital belly of occipitofrontalis	17 Parotid gland	28 Levator anguli oris
	18 Masseter	29 Facial artery
	19 Marginal mandibular branch of facial nerve	30 Depressor anguli oris
	20 Buccal branch of facial nerve	31 Mentalis

Face, superficial structures II – *from the left*

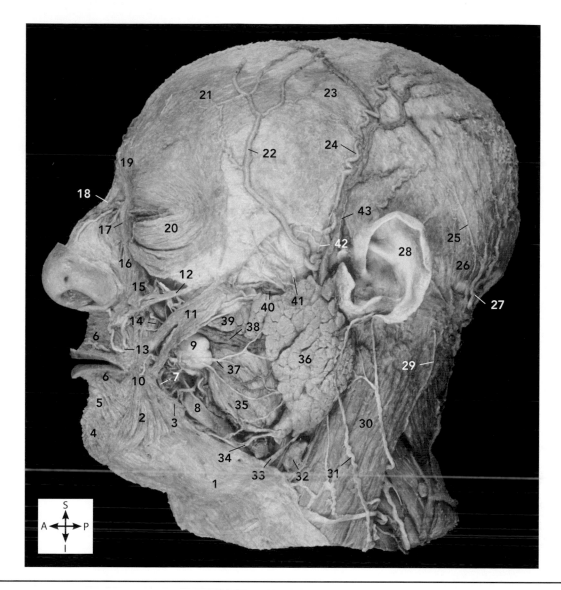

1	Platysma	
2	Depressor anguli oris	
3	Risorius	
4	Mentalis	
5	Depressor labii inferioris	
6	Orbicularis oris	
7	Facial artery	
8	Facial vein	
9	Buccal fat pad	
10	Modiolus	
11	Zygomaticus major	
12	Zygomaticus minor	
13	Superior labial artery	
14	Levator anguli oris	
15	Levator labii superioris	
16	Levator labii superioris alaeque nasi	
17	Nasalis	
18	Procerus	
19	Depressor supercilii	
20	Orbicularis oculi	
21	Frontal belly of occipitofrontalis	
22	Frontal branch of superficial temporal artery	
23	Epicranial aponeurosis	
24	Parietal branch of superficial temporal artery	
25	Greater occipital nerve	
26	Occipital belly of occipitofrontalis	
27	Occipital artery and vein	
28	Cartilage of auricle (pinna)	
29	Lesser occipital nerve	
30	Sternocleidomastoid	
31	Great auricular nerve	
32	Cervical lymph node	
33	Cervical branch of facial nerve	
34	Marginal mandibular branch of facial nerve	
35	Masseter	
36	Parotid gland	
37	Buccal branch of facial nerve	
38	Parotid duct	
39	Accessory parotid gland	
40	Transverse facial artery	
41	Zygomatic branches of facial nerve	
42	Temporal branches of facial nerve	
43	Auriculotemporal nerve	

Masticatory muscles I – *from the left*

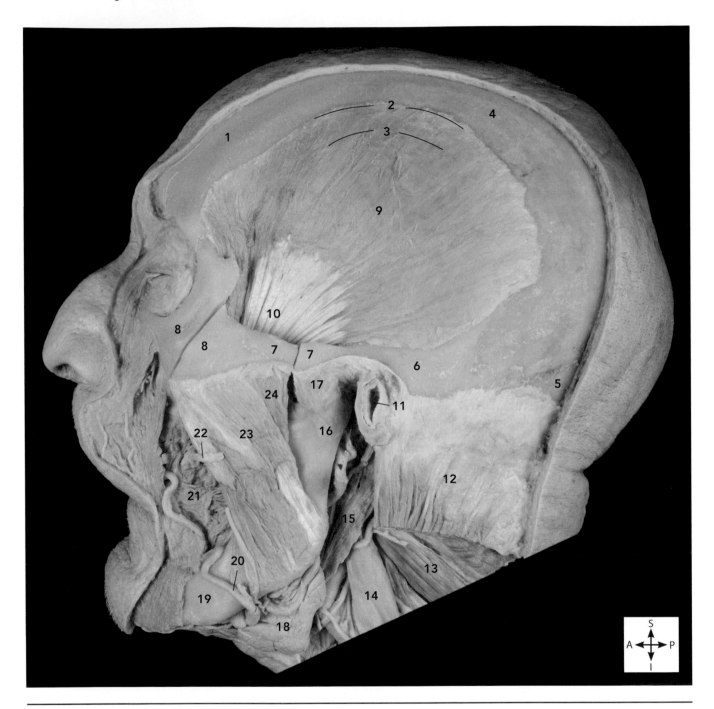

1 Frontal bone	9 Temporalis muscle	17 Lateral ligament of temporomandibular joint
2 Superior ⎤ temporal line	10 Temporalis tendon	18 Submandibular gland
3 Inferior ⎦	11 External acoustic meatus	19 Body of mandible
4 Parietal bone	12 Sternocleidomastoid	20 Facial artery
5 Occipital bone	13 Levator scapulae	21 Buccinator
6 Temporal bone	14 Internal jugular vein	22 Parotid duct
7 Zygomatic process of temporal bone	15 Posterior belly of digastric	23 Superficial ⎤ part of masseter
8 Zygomatic bone	16 Neck of mandible	24 Deep ⎦

Masticatory muscles II, with masseter reflected inferiorly to display temporalis insertion – *from the left*

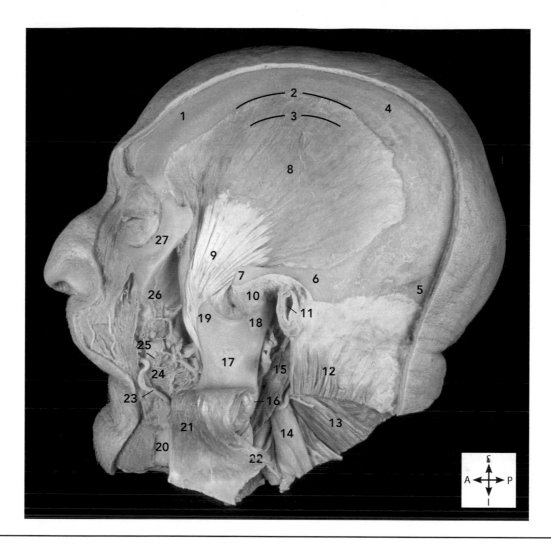

1	Frontal bone	11	External acoustic meatus	23	Facial artery
2	Superior ⌉ temporal line	12	Sternocleidomastoid	24	Buccinator
3	Inferior ⌋	13	Levator scapulae	25	Parotid duct
4	Parietal bone	14	Internal jugular vein	26	Infratemporal surface of maxilla
5	Occipital bone	15	Posterior belly of digastric	27	Zygomatic bone
6	Temporal bone	16	Angle ⌉		
7	Zygomatic process of temporal bone	17	Ramus		
8	Temporalis muscle	18	Neck	of mandible	
9	Temporalis tendon	19	Coronoid process		
10	Lateral ligament of temporomandibular joint	20	Body ⌋		
		21	Superficial ⌉ inner part		
		22	Deep ⌋ of masseter		

The masticatory muscles are:

➤ Temporalis, masseter, medial and lateral pterygoid.

Insertion of temporalis tendon:

➤ Is to the apex, anterior and posterior borders and medial surface of the coronoid process of the mandible, extending down the anterior border of the ramus near to the third molar tooth.

Infratemporal fossa I, with partial reduction of the mandible and exposure of the mandibular canal – *from the left*

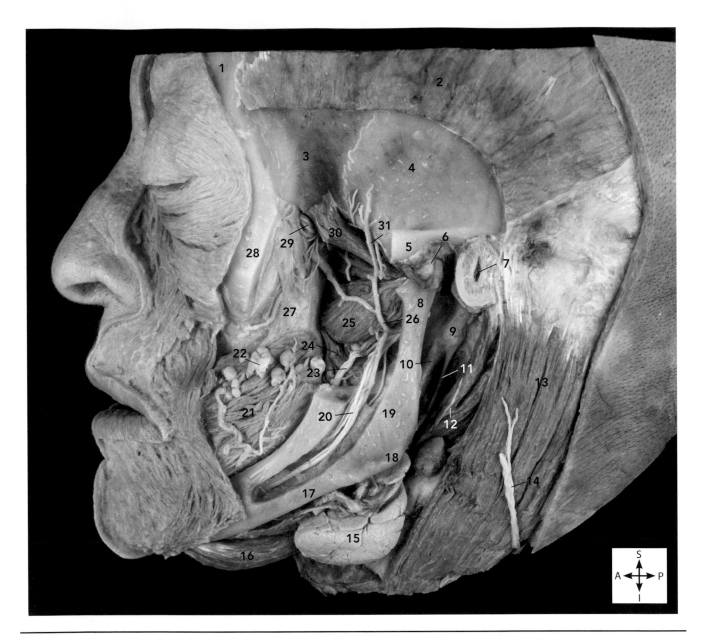

1	Frontal bone	11	Stylohyoid ligament	23	Lingual nerve
2	Temporalis	12	Posterior belly of digastric	24	Medial pterygoid
3	Greater wing of sphenoid	13	Sternocleidomastoid	25	Lower head of lateral pterygoid
4	Squamous part of temporal bone	14	Great auricular nerve	26	Maxillary artery
5	Zygomatic process of temporal bone	15	Submandibular gland	27	Infratemporal surface of maxilla
6	Capsule of temporomandibular joint	16	Anterior belly of digastric	28	Orbital margin of zygomatic bone
7	External acoustic meatus	17	Base / 18 Angle / 19 Ramus ⎤ of mandible	29	Maxillary nerve
8	Neck of mandible	20	Inferior alveolar nerve and artery within mandibular canal	30	Upper head of lateral pterygoid
9	Styloid process	21	Buccinator	31	Deep temporal artery
10	Styloglossus	22	Parotid duct		

Infratemporal fossa II, larynx and deep neck, with removal of the majority of the mandible – *from the left*

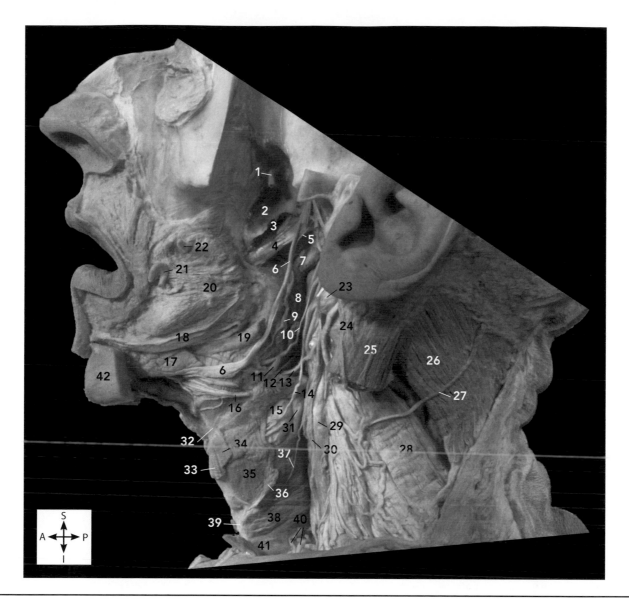

1	Maxillary artery entering pterygomaxillary fissure	
2	Lateral pterygoid plate of sphenoid	
3	Tensor veli palatini	
4	Levator veli palatini	
5	Chorda tympani	
6	Lingual nerve	
7	Pharyngobasilar fascia	
8	Superior constrictor of pharynx	
9	Ascending palatine artery	
10	Glossopharyngeal nerve	
11	Stylohyoid ligament	
12	Middle constrictor of pharynx	
13	Lingual artery	
14	Internal laryngeal nerve	
15	Thyrohyoid membrane	
16	Hypoglossal nerve	
17	Sublingual gland	
18	Mucoperiosteum of mandible	
19	Styloglossus	
20	Buccinator	
21	Facial artery	
22	Parotid duct	
23	Internal jugular vein	
24	Occipital artery	
25	Sternocleidomastoid	
26	Splenius capitis	
27	Lesser occipital nerve	
28	Levator scapulae	
29	Vagus nerve	
30	Sympathetic trunk	
31	Superior horn of thyroid cartilage	
32	Body of hyoid bone	
33	Sternohyoid	
34	Superior belly of omohyoid	
35	Thyrohyoid	
36	Sternothyroid	
37	External laryngeal nerve	
38	Cricothyroid	
39	Arch of cricoid cartilage	
40	Recurrent laryngeal nerve	
41	Trachea	
42	Body of mandible	

Submandibular region and larynx – *from the left*

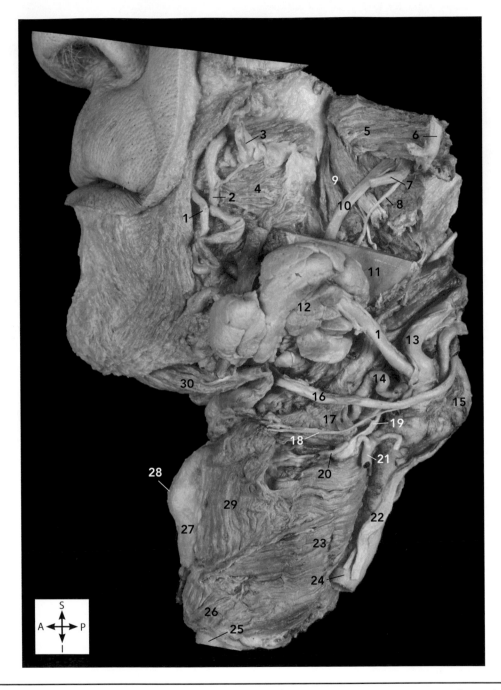

1	Facial artery	11	Ramus of mandible	21	Superior thyroid artery
2	Facial vein	12	Submandibular gland (reflected superiorly)	22	Vagus nerve
3	Parotid duct	13	External carotid artery	23	Inferior constrictor of pharynx
4	Buccinator	14	Lingual artery	24	Common carotid artery
5	Lower head of lateral pterygoid	15	Internal carotid artery	25	Trachea
6	Maxillary artery	16	Hypoglossal nerve	26	Cricothyroid
7	Inferior alveolar nerve	17	Stylohyoid	27	Lamina of thyroid cartilage
8	Nerve to mylohyoid	18	Nerve to thyrohyoid	28	Laryngeal prominence of thyroid cartilage
9	Medial pterygoid	19	Internal laryngeal nerve	29	Thyrohyoid
10	Lingual nerve	20	Superior laryngeal artery	30	Anterior belly of digastric

A Larynx – *from the front*

B Larynx – *from behind*

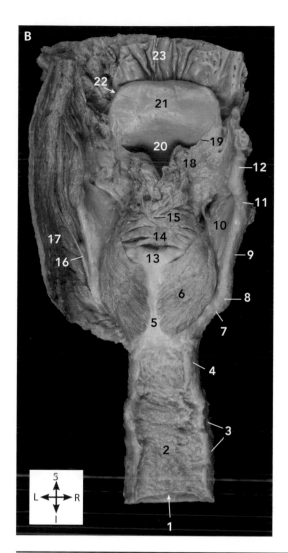

A

1 Trachea
2 First tracheal cartilage
3 Arch of cricoid cartilage
4 Cricothyroid (straight part)
5 Conus elasticus (cricovocal membrane)
6 Cricothyroid ligament
7 Cricothyroid joint
8 Inferior horn of thyroid cartilage
9 Lamina of thyroid cartilage
10 Laryngeal prominence of thyroid cartilage
11 Thyrohyoid membrane
12 Superior horn of thyroid cartilage
13 Body of hyoid bone
14 Omohyoid and sternohyoid (reflected superiorly)
15 Posterior wall of oropharynx
16 Thyrohyoid
17 Inferior constrictor of pharynx

1 Trachea
2 Trachealis
3 Tracheal cartilages
4 First tracheal cartilage
5 Site of attachment of oesophageal tendon
6 Posterior crico-arytenoid
7 Cricothyroid joint
8 Inferior horn of thyroid cartilage
9 Lamina of thyroid cartilage
10 Piriform recess
11 Superior horn of thyroid cartilage
12 Greater horn of hyoid bone

13 Lamina of cricoid cartilage
14 Transverse arytenoid
15 Oblique arytenoid
16 Recurrent laryngeal nerve
17 Inferior constrictor of pharynx
18 Aryepiglotticus
19 Aryepiglottic fold
20 Vestibule
21 Epiglottis
22 Vallecula
23 Dorsum of tongue

Hyoid bone and cartilages of the larynx – *A from the front; B from behind*

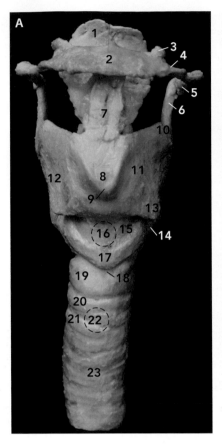

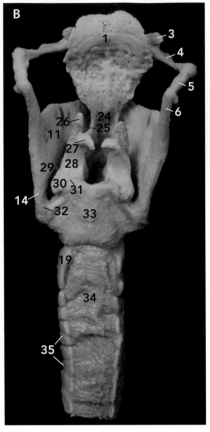

1	Epiglottic cartilage	15	Cricothyroid ligament	27	Corniculate cartilage

1 Epiglottic cartilage
2 Body of hyoid bone
3 Lesser horn ⎤
4 Greater horn ⎦ of hyoid bone
5 Lateral thyrohyoid ligament
6 Superior horn of thyroid cartilage
7 Thyrohyoid membrane
8 Thyroid notch
9 Laryngeal prominence ⎤
10 Superior tubercle
11 Lamina   of thyroid
12 Oblique line   cartilage
13 Inferior tubercle
14 Inferior horn ⎦

15 Cricothyroid ligament
16 Circled – site for inferior laryngotomy
17 Arch of cricoid cartilage
18 Cricotracheal ligament
19 First ⎤
20 Second   tracheal
21 Third   cartilage ⎦
22 Circled – site for tracheotomy
23 Trachea
24 Thyroepiglottic ligament
25 Vestibular fold
26 Cuneiform cartilage

27 Corniculate cartilage
28 Arytenoid cartilage
29 Piriform recess
30 Muscular process of arytenoid cartilage
31 Crico-arytenoid joint
32 Cricothyroid joint
33 Lamina of cricoid cartilage
34 Trachealis
35 Tracheal cartilages

The hyoid bone:
➤ Body and greater horns are palpable in the neck at the level of the third (CIII) cervical vertebra.

The lamina of the thyroid cartilage:
➤ Form the laryngeal prominence in the middle of the front of the neck, more obvious in males than females, hence the common term for it (Adam's apple); it is palpable at the level of the fourth (CIV) and the fifth (CV) cervical vertebra.

The arch of the cricoid cartilage:
➤ Can be located and palpated approximately 5 cm above the sternocostal notch at the level of the sixth (CVI) cervical vertebra.

Pharynx posterior surface – *from behind*

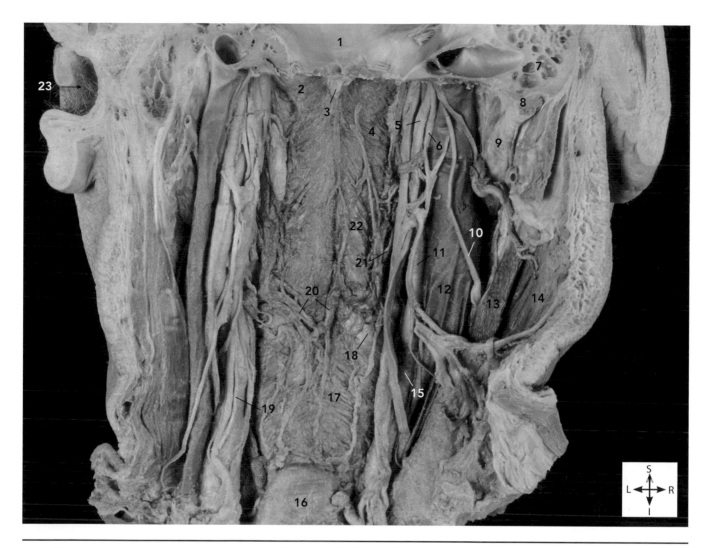

1	Clivus	
2	Pharyngobasilar fascia	
3	Attachment of the pharyngeal raphae to the pharyngeal tubercle of the base of the skull	
4	Superior constrictor of pharynx	
5	Vagus nerve	
6	Hypoglossal nerve	
7	Mastoid air cells	
8	Mastoid process of temporal bone	

9	Posterior belly of digastric
10	Accessory nerve
11	Internal carotid artery
12	Internal jugular vein
13	Sternocleidomastoid
14	Trapezius
15	Common carotid artery
16	Cricopharyngeal ⎤ part of inferior
17	Thyropharyngeal ⎦ constrictor of pharynx
18	Tip of greater horn of hyoid bone
19	Sympathetic trunk

20	Pharyngeal veins
21	Ascending pharyngeal artery
22	Middle constrictor of pharynx
23	External acoustic meatus

The pharyngeal plexus of nerves and veins:
➤ Are mostly located on the posterior surface of the middle constrictor muscle.
➤ The plexus of nerves is formed by the pharyngeal branches of both the glossopharyngeal (IX) and vagus (X) nerves.
➤ The glossopharyngeal component is afferent only.
➤ The vagal component is motor to the pharynx and palate as well as containing afferent fibres.

Adult skull, anterior external base, dentition – *from below*

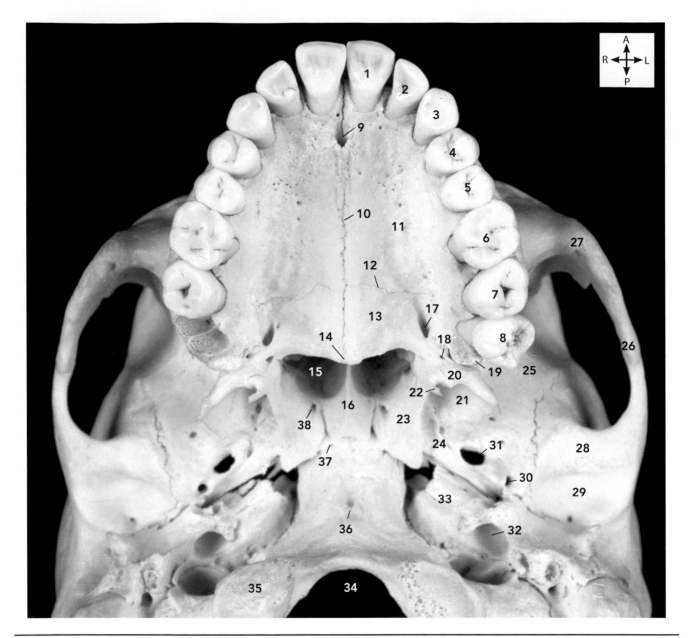

1 Central ⎤ incisor	14 Posterior nasal spine	27 Zygomatic bone
2 Lateral ⎦	15 Posterior nasal aperture	28 Articular tubercle
3 Canine	16 Vomer	29 Mandibular fossa
4 First ⎤ premolar	17 Greater palatine foramen	30 Foramen spinosum
5 Second ⎦	18 Lesser palatine foramina	31 Foramen ovale
6 First ⎤	19 Tuberosity of maxilla	32 Carotid canal
7 Second ⎥ molar	20 Pyramidal process of maxilla	33 Apex of petrous part of
8 Third ⎦	21 Lateral pterygoid plate	temporal bone
9 Incisive foramen	22 Pterygoid hamulus	34 Foramen magnum
10 Median palatine suture	23 Medial pterygoid plate	35 Occipital condyle
11 Palatine process of maxilla	24 Scaphoid fossa	36 Pharyngeal tubercle
12 Transverse palatine suture	25 Infratemporal crest	37 Vomerovaginal canal
13 Horizontal plate of palatine bone	26 Zygomatic process of temporal bone	38 Palatovaginal canal

Adult mandible, dentition – *from above*

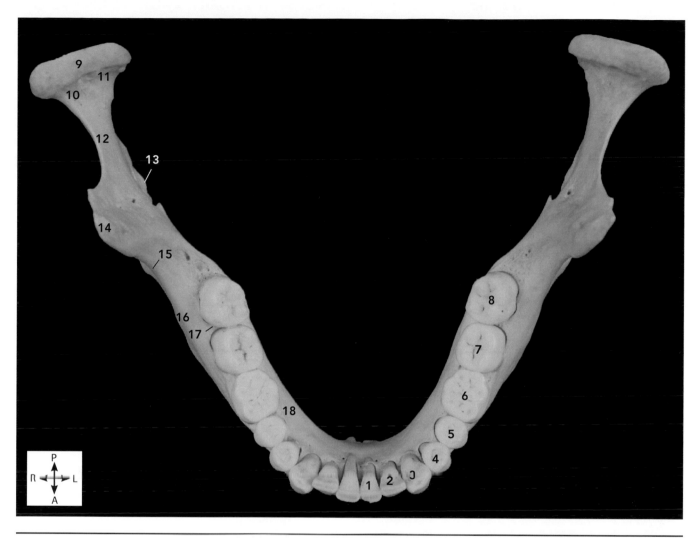

1	Central	incisor	8	Third molar	15	Anterior border of ramus and coronoid notch
2	Lateral		9	Head — forming condylar	16	Body of mandible
3	Canine		10	Neck — process of mandible	17	Alveolar part
4	First	premolar	11	Pterygoid fovea	18	Sublingual fossa
5	Second		12	Mandibular notch		
6	First	molar	13	Angle — process of		
7	Second		14	Coronoid — mandible		

Normal eruption times for teeth are:

➤ Deciduous teeth:
- Lower lateral incisors – 6 months
- Upper central incisors – 7 months
- Upper lateral incisors – 8 months
- Lower lateral incisors – 9 months
- First molars – 12 months
- Canines – 18 months
- Second molars – 24 months

➤ Permanent teeth:
- First permanent molars – 6 years
- Central incisors – 7 years
- Lateral incisors – 8 years
- First premolars – 9 years
- Second premolars – 10 years
- Canines – 11 years
- Second permanent molars – 12 years
- Third permanent molars (wisdom teeth) –18 years

A Mouth and pharynx, paramedian sagittal section – *from the right*

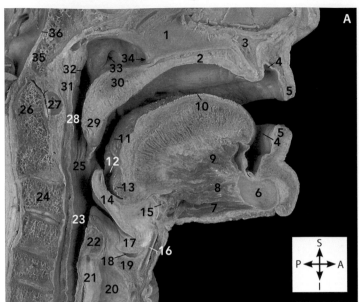

B Structures of the tongue exposed in a paramedian sagittal section – *from the right*

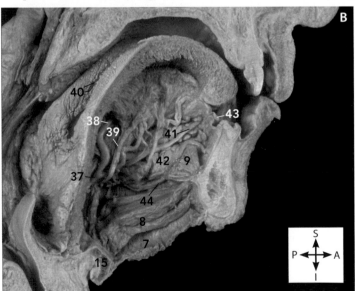

C Isolated left sublingual gland, actual size as presented at dissection – *from the right*

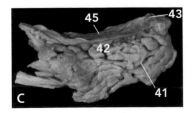

1 Nasal septum
2 Hard palate
3 Maxilla
4 Vestibule of mouth
5 Lip
6 Body of mandible
7 Mylohyoid
8 Geniohyoid
9 Genioglossus
10 Presulcal ⎤ part of dorsum
11 Postsulcal ⎦ of tongue
12 Vallecula
13 Lingual tonsil
14 Epiglottis
15 Body of hyoid bone
16 Lamina of thyroid cartilage
17 Vestibular fold
18 Ventricle of larynx
19 Vocal fold (vocal cord)
20 Lower part of larynx
21 Lamina of cricoid cartilage
22 Transverse arytenoid
23 Laryngopharynx (laryngeal part of pharynx)
24 Body of third (CIII) cervical vertebra
25 Oropharynx (oral part of pharynx)
26 Dens of axis (second [CII] cervical vertebra)
27 Anterior arch of atlas (first [CI] cervical vertebra)
28 Nasal part of pharynx (nasopharynx)
29 Uvula
30 Soft palate
31 Pharyngeal tonsil
32 Pharyngeal recess
33 Opening of auditory tube
34 Posterior nasal aperture
35 Anterior margin of foramen magnum
36 Clivus
37 Lingual artery
38 Deep lingual artery
39 Lingual nerve
40 Fungiform papillae
41 Submandibular gland
42 Sublingual duct
43 Orifice of submandibular duct on sublingual papilla
44 Sublingual artery
45 Mucous membrane

Floor of mouth, deep and adjacent structures exposed in a paramedian sagittal section – *from the right*

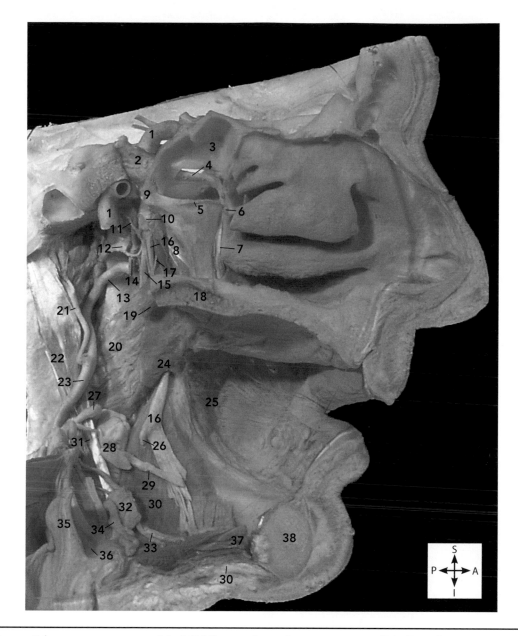

1	Internal carotid artery	14	Middle meningeal artery	27	Facial artery
2	Trigeminal ganglia	15	Inferior alveolar nerve	28	Deep part of submandibular gland
3	Sphenoidal sinus	16	Lingual nerve	29	Submandibular duct
4	Maxillary nerve	17	Nerve to medial pterygoid	30	Mylohyoid
5	Nerve of pterygoid canal	18	Soft palate	31	Tendon of digastric
6	Pterygopalatine ganglia	19	Palatopharyngeus	32	Hyoglossus
7	Greater palatine nerve	20	Medial pterygoid	33	Hypoglossal nerve
8	Tensor veli palatine	21	Occipital artery	34	Lingual artery
9	Mandibular nerve	22	Posterior belly of digastric	35	Epiglottis
10	Otic ganglion	23	External carotid artery	36	Vallecula
11	Chorda tympani	24	Superior constrictor of pharynx	37	Geniohyoid
12	Auriculotemporal nerve	25	Buccinator	38	Body of mandible
13	Maxillary artery	26	Submandibular ganglion		

A Nasal septum, paramedian sagittal section – *from the right*

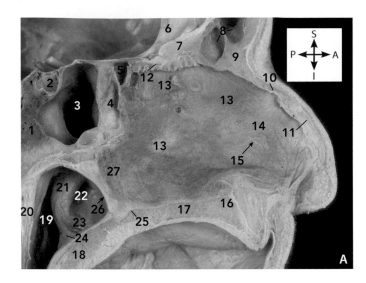

1 Sphenoid
2 Pituitary gland
3 Sphenoidal sinus
4 Spheno-ethmoidal recess
5 Ethmoidal air cell
6 Falx cerebri
7 Crista galli of ethmoid bone
8 Frontal sinus
9 Frontal bone
10 Nasal bone
11 Lateral nasal cartilage
12 Cribriform plate of ethmoid bone
13 Perpendicular plate of ethmoid bone
14 Septal cartilage
15 Vomeronasal organ
16 Nasal crest of maxilla
17 Hard palate
18 Soft palate
19 Pharyngeal recess
20 Pharyngeal tonsil
21 Tubal elevation
22 Opening of auditory tube
23 Levator elevation
24 Salpingopharyngeal fold
25 Nasal crest of palatine bone
26 Posterior nasal aperture
27 Vomer

B With partial removal of the cribriform plate of the ethmoid bone and nasal septum to expose the mucosal lining – *from the right*

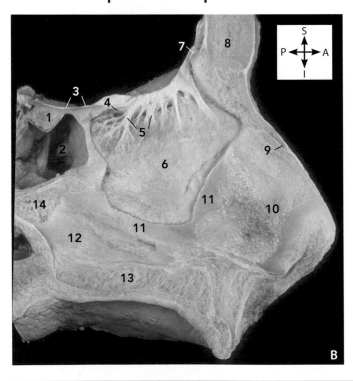

1 Pituitary gland
2 Sphenoidal sinus
3 Dural lining of anterior cranial fossa
4 Cribriform plate of ethmoid bone
5 Dural sheaths containing fine filaments of olfactory nerves (I) within dural sheaths invaginating foramina within the cribriform plate of ethmoid bone
6 Mucous membrane lining of nasal septum
7 Crista galli of ethmoid bone
8 Frontal bone
9 Nasal bone
10 Septal cartilage
11 Perpendicular plate of ethmoid bone
12 Vomer
13 Hard palate
14 Sphenoid

Damage and interruption of the olfactory nerve filaments:
➤ May occur following a head injury and in particular fractures of the anterior cranial fossa.
➤ Such an injury may present as rhinorrhoea due to leakage of cerebrospinal fluid (CSF) from the ruptured dural sheaths within the cribriform plate of the ethmoid bone

A Lateral wall of the nasal cavity and nasopharynx, paramedian sagittal section with removal of the nasal septum – *from the right*

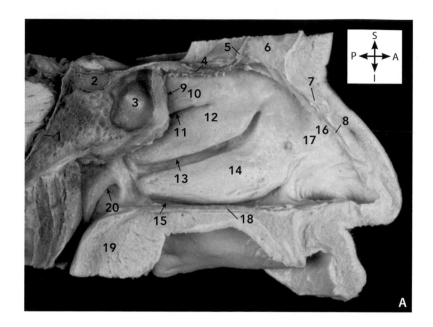

1 Clivus	10 Superior nasal concha
2 Pituitary gland	11 Superior meatus
3 Sphenoidal sinus	12 Middle nasal concha
4 Cribriform plate of ethmoid bone	13 Middle meatus
5 Crista galli of ethmoid bone	14 Inferior nasal concha
6 Frontal bone	15 Inferior meatus
7 Nasal bone	16 Atrium
8 Nasal cartilage	17 Agger nasi
9 Spheno-ethmoidal recess	18 Hard palate
	19 Soft palate
	20 Opening of auditory tube

B Semilunar hiatus, with extensive removal of the superior and middle nasal conchae – *from the right*

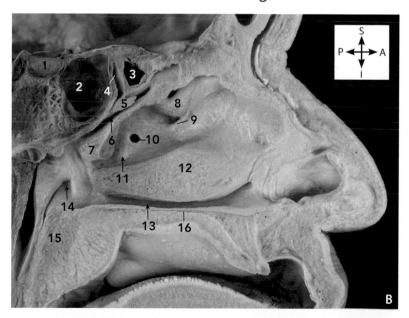

1 Pituitary gland	8 Ethmoidal bulla
2 Sphenoidal sinus	9 Semilunar hiatus
3 Ethmoidal air cell	10 Aperture of maxillary sinus
4 Spheno-ethmoidal recess	11 Middle meatus
5 Base of superior nasal concha	12 Inferior nasal concha
6 Superior meatus	13 Inferior meatus
7 Middle nasal concha	14 Opening of auditory tube
	15 Soft palate
	16 Hard palate

There are four pairs of paranasal sinuses:
➤ The left and right of each pair, are rarely truly symmetrical and can vary considerably in both shape and size.
➤ **Frontal** – two in the lower part of the squamous part of the frontal bone.
➤ **Ethmoidal** – two in the body of the ethmoid bone, divided by bony septa into a number of ethmoidal air cells.
➤ **Sphenoidal** – in the body of the sphenoid.
➤ **Maxillary** – in the body of the maxilla.

A Lateral wall of the nasal cavity, paramedian sagittal section with removal of the nasal septum and a portion of inferior nasal concha to display the opening of the nasolacrimal duct – *from the right*

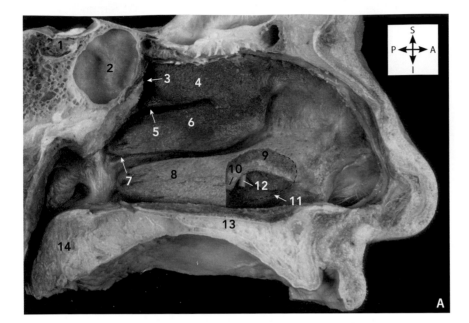

1 Pituitary gland
2 Sphenoidal sinus
3 Spheno-ethmoidal recess
4 Superior nasal concha
5 Superior meatus
6 Middle nasal concha
7 Middle meatus
8 Inferior nasal concha
9 Mucosa ⎤ of inferior
10 Bone ⎦ nasal concha
11 Inferior meatus
12 Blue marker in opening of nasolacrimal duct
13 Hard ⎤ palate
14 Soft ⎦

B With removal of a posterior portion of the nasal conchae to expose the palatine canal – *from the right*

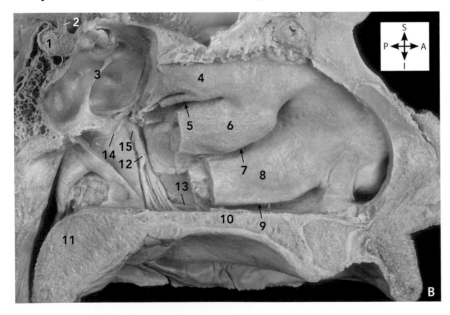

1 Pituitary gland
2 Infundibulum
3 Sphenoidal sinus
4 Superior nasal concha
5 Superior meatus
6 Middle nasal concha
7 Middle meatus
8 Inferior nasal concha
9 Inferior meatus
10 Hard palate
11 Soft palate
12 Greater palatine nerve in palatine canal
13 Posterior inferior nasal nerve
14 Lateral posterior nasal nerve
15 Pterygopalatine ganglion

Drainage into the meatus:
➤ **Spheno-ethmoidal recess** – from the sphenoidal sinus.
➤ **Superior meatus** – from the posterior ethmoidal air cells.
➤ **Middle meatus** – from the frontal sinus, anterior and middle ethmoidal air cells and the maxillary sinus.
➤ **Inferior meatus** – from the nasolacrimal duct.

Structures of the external nose – *A, B from the left; C from the front*

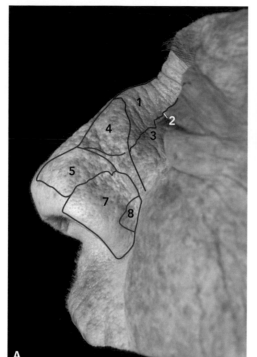

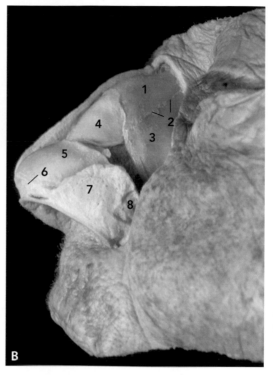

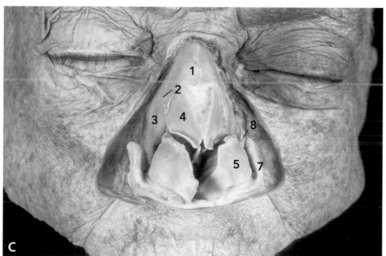

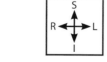

1 Nasal bone
2 Nasomaxillary suture
3 Frontal process of maxilla
4 Lateral nasal cartilage

5 Greater nasal cartilage
6 Septal process (medial crus) of
   greater nasal cartilage

7 Fibrofatty tissue
8 Lesser alar cartilage

The nose:
➤ The main parts forming and giving shape to this distinct individual facial structure are:
 • **Externally** – the two nasal bones and the lateral, greater and lesser nasal cartilages.
 • **Internally** – the nasal septum, which has three main parts to its form, the bony vomer, perpendicular plate of the ethmoid bone and pliable nasal cartilage.
➤ A common occurrence is for the septum to deviate to one side of the nasal cavity and in so doing can cause sufficient obstruction to compromise the drainage of the nose and inspiration.

Adult skull, structures relating to the orbit – *from the front right and slightly above*

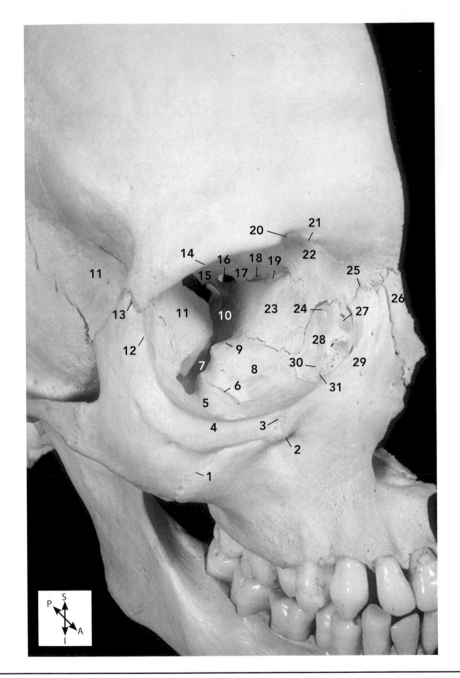

1	Zygomaticomaxillary suture	11	Greater wing of sphenoid	22	Orbital part of frontal bone
2	Infra-orbital foramen	12	Tubercle of zygomatic bone	23	Orbital plate of ethmoid bone
3	Zygomaticomaxillary foramen	13	Frontozygomatic suture	24	Posterior lacrimal crest
4	Infra-orbital margin	14	Supra-orbital margin	25	Frontomaxillary suture
5	Orbital surface of zygomatic bone	15	Lesser wing of sphenoid	26	Nasal bone
6	Infra-orbital groove	16	Optic canal	27	Fossa for lacrimal sac
7	Inferior orbital fissure	17	Body of sphenoid	28	Lacrimal bone
8	Orbital surface of maxilla	18	Posterior ⎤ ethmoidal	29	Frontal process of maxilla
9	Orbital process of palatine bone	19	Anterior ⎦ foramen	30	Lacrimal groove
10	Superior orbital foramen	20	Supra-orbital foramen	31	Anterior lacrimal crest
		21	Frontal notch		

Adult skull, with coloured bones – *from the front left and slightly above*

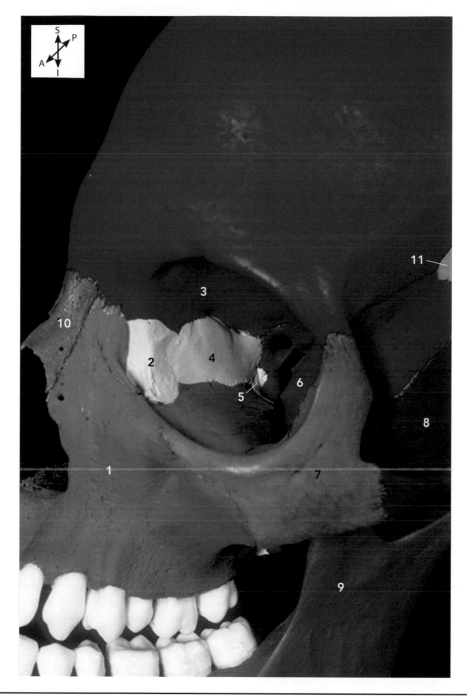

1	Maxilla	5	Palatine bone	9	Mandible
2	Lacrimal bone	6	Sphenoid	10	Nasal bone
3	Frontal bone	7	Zygomatic bone	11	Parietal bone
4	Ethmoid bone	8	Temporal bone		

Bones forming the orbit:
➤ **Roof** – orbital part of the frontal bone and lesser wing of sphenoid.
➤ **Lateral wall** – orbital surfaces of the greater wing of the sphenoid and the zygomatic bone.
➤ **Floor** – orbital surfaces of the maxilla and the zygomatic bone with orbital process of the palatine bone.
➤ **Medial wall** – frontal process of the maxilla, lacrimal bone, orbital plate of the ethmoid bone and body of the sphenoid.

A Left orbit with roof removed – *from above*

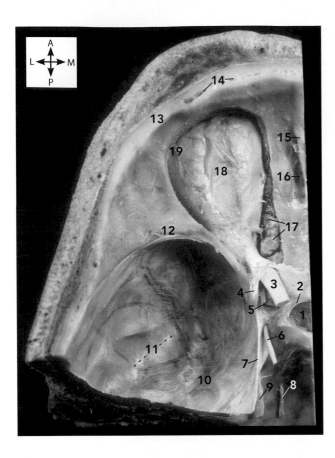

1	Pituitary gland
2	Diaphragma sellae
3	Optic nerve (II)
4	Anterior clinoid process
5	Internal carotid artery
6	Oculomotor nerve (III)
7	Free margin of tentorium cerebelli
8	Abducent nerve (VI)
9	Trigeminal nerve (V)
10	Tentorium cerebelli
11	Attached margin of tentorium cerebelli
12	Posterior margin of lesser wing of sphenoid
13	Frontal bone
14	Frontal sinus
15	Crista galli of ethmoid bone
16	Cribriform plate of ethmoid bone
17	Ethmoidal air cells
18	Orbital fat
19	Lacrimal gland

B Superficial structures – *from above*

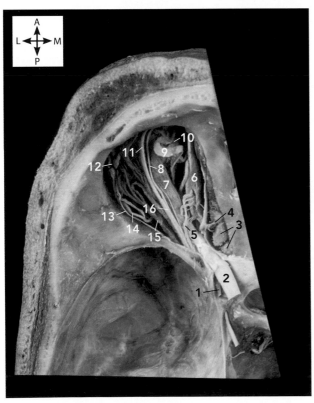

1	Internal carotid artery
2	Optic nerve (II)
3	Ethmoidal air cells
4	Posterior ethmoidal artery
5	Trochlear nerve
6	Superior oblique
7	Levator palpebrae superioris
8	Supratrochlear nerve
9	Superior ophthalmic vein
10	Trochlea
11	Supra-orbital nerve
12	Lacrimal gland
13	Lacrimal nerve
14	Lacrimal artery
15	Lateral rectus
16	Frontal nerve

Left orbit with roof and lateral wall removed – *from above left and slightly behind*

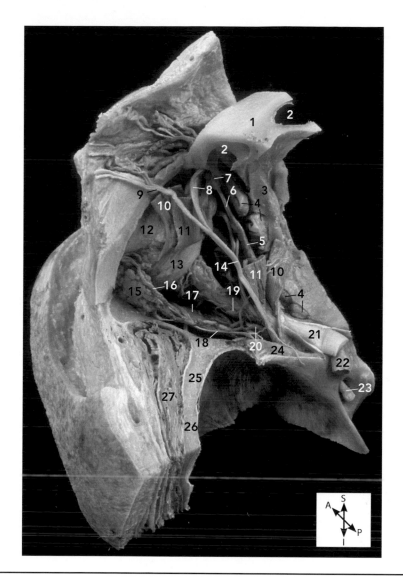

1	Frontal bone	11	Superior rectus (bisected and reflected superiorly)	21	Optic nerve (II)
2	Frontal sinus			22	Internal carotid artery
3	Crista galli of ethmoid bone	12	Superior ⎤ outer surface	23	Oculomotor nerve (III)
4	Ethmoidal air cells	13	Posterior ⎦ of eyeball	24	Lesser ⎤ wing of sphenoid
5	Superior oblique	14	Frontal nerve	25	Greater ⎦
6	Tendon of superior oblique	15	Lacrimal gland	26	Temporal bone
7	Trochlea	16	Lacrimal artery	27	Temporalis
8	Supratrochlear nerve	17	Lateral rectus		
9	Supra-orbital nerve	18	Lacrimal nerve		
10	Levator palpebrae superioris (bisected and reflected superiorly)	19	Ciliary ganglion		
		20	Ophthalmic artery		

Muscles responsible for movements of the eye:
➤ **Inwards** – superior rectus, medial rectus and inferior rectus.
➤ **Outwards** – lateral rectus, superior oblique and inferior oblique.
➤ **Upwards** – depends upon both the superior rectus and inferior oblique.
➤ **Downwards** – depends upon both the inferior rectus and superior oblique.

Left orbit with partial removal of roof and lateral wall – *from the left*

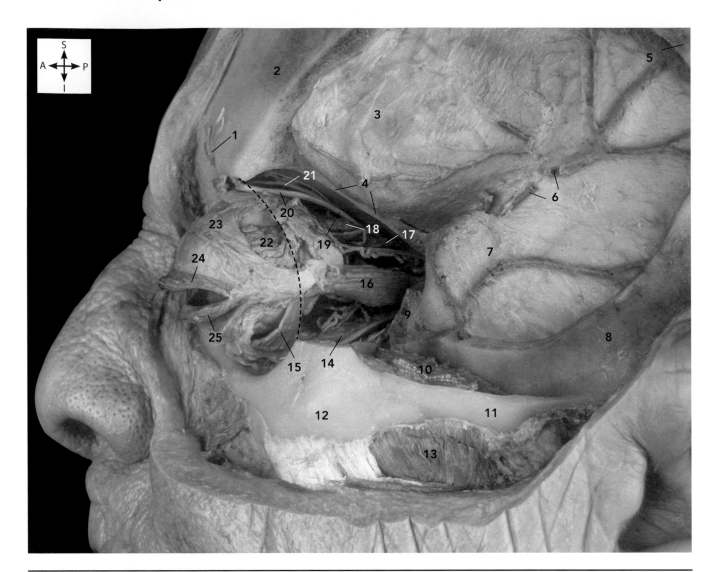

1	Supra-orbital nerve emerging from supra-orbital notch	8 Temporal bone
2	Frontal bone	9 Greater wing of sphenoid
3	Dura mater overlying frontal lobe of cerebral hemisphere	10 Temporalis
4	Orbital part of frontal bone	11 Zygomatic process of temporal bone
5	Parietal bone	12 Zygomatic bone
6	Frontal branch of middle meningeal artery	13 Masseter
7	Dura mater overlying temporal lobe of cerebral hemisphere	14 Inferior rectus
		15 Inferior oblique
		16 Lateral rectus

1 Supra-orbital nerve emerging from supra-orbital notch
2 Frontal bone
3 Dura mater overlying frontal lobe of cerebral hemisphere
4 Orbital part of frontal bone
5 Parietal bone
6 Frontal branch of middle meningeal artery
7 Dura mater overlying temporal lobe of cerebral hemisphere

8 Temporal bone
9 Greater wing of sphenoid
10 Temporalis
11 Zygomatic process of temporal bone
12 Zygomatic bone
13 Masseter
14 Inferior rectus
15 Inferior oblique
16 Lateral rectus

17 Superior rectus
18 Levator palpebrae superioris
19 Frontal nerve
20 Supra-orbital nerve
21 Supratrochlear nerve
22 Lacrimal gland
23 Aponeurosis of levator palpebrae superioris
24 Upper ⎤ eyelid
25 Lower ⎦

Left orbit with partial removal of roof and lateral wall – *from the left*

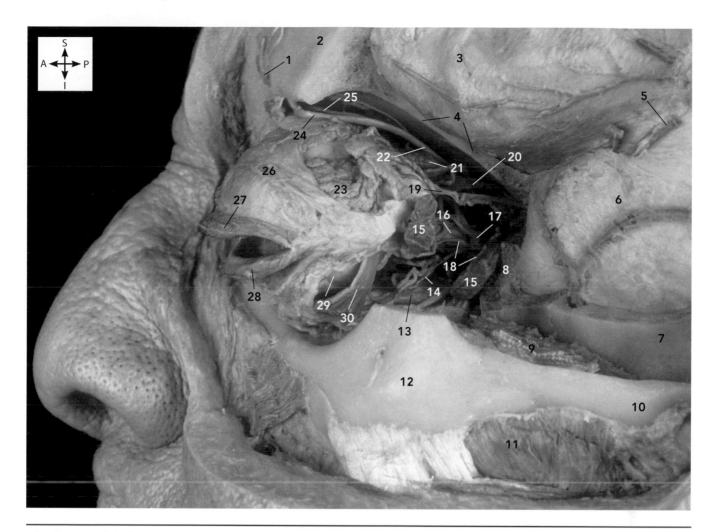

1   Supra orbital nerve emerging from supra-orbital notch
2   Frontal bone
3   Dura mater overlying frontal lobe of cerebral hemisphere
4   Orbital part of frontal bone
5   Frontal branch of middle meningeal artery
6   Dura mater overlying temporal lobe of cerebral hemisphere
7   Temporal bone
8   Greater wing of sphenoid
9   Temporalis
10 Zygomatic process of temporal bone
11 Masseter
12 Zygomatic bone
13 Inferior rectus
14 Nerve to inferior rectus
15 Lateral rectus (divided and reflected laterally)
16 Optic nerve
17 Ciliary ganglion
18 Short ciliary nerves
19 Lacrimal artery, vein and nerve
20 Superior rectus
21 Levator palpebrae superioris
22 Frontal nerve
23 Lacrimal gland
24 Supra-orbital nerve
25 Supratrochlear nerve
26 Aponeurosis of levator palpebrae superioris
27 Upper ⎤ eyelid
28 Lower ⎦ eyelid
29 Inferior outer surface of eyeball
30 Inferior oblique

Left orbit with eyeball removed – *from the front*

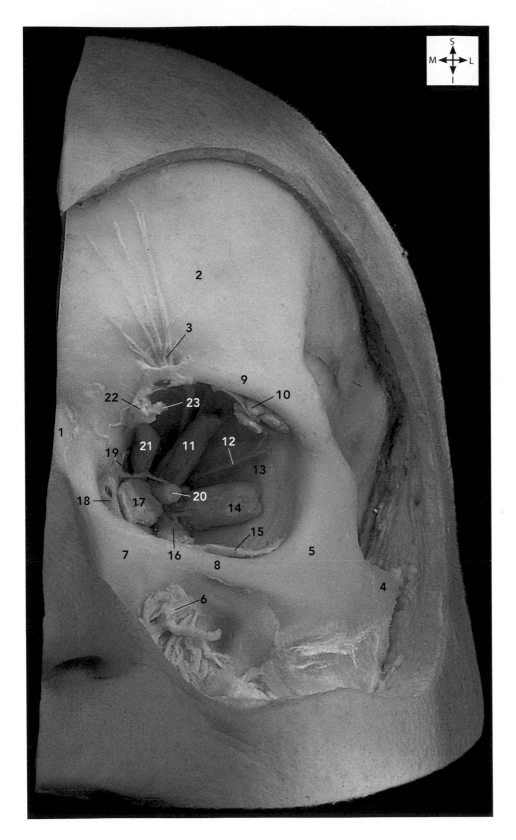

1 Nasal bone
2 Frontal bone
3 Supra-orbital nerve emerging from supra-orbital foramen
4 Zygomatic process of temporal bone
5 Zygomatic bone
6 Infra-orbital nerve emerging from infra-orbital foramen
7 Maxilla
8 Infra-orbital ⎤
9 Supra-orbital ⎦ margin
10 Lacrimal gland
11 Superior rectus
12 Lacrimal nerve
13 Greater wing of sphenoid
14 Lateral rectus
15 Inferior oblique
16 Inferior ⎤
17 Medial ⎦ rectus
18 Lacrimal sac
19 Nasociliary nerve
20 Optic nerve
21 Superior oblique
22 Trochlea
23 Tendon of superior oblique

A Left orbit and nasolacrimal duct – *from the front and slightly left*

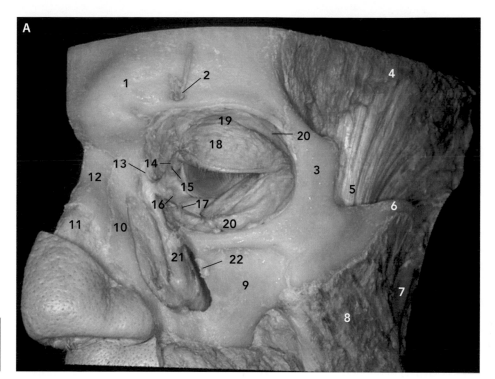

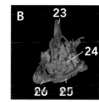

B Isolated left lacrimal gland, actual size as presented at dissection – *from above*

1	Frontal bone
2	Supra-orbital artery and nerve emerging from supra-orbital notch
3	Zygomatic bone
4	Temporalis muscle
5	Temporalis tendon
6	Zygomatic process of temporal bone
7	Ramus of mandible
8	Masseter
9	Maxilla
10	Frontal process of maxilla
11	Nasal cartilage
12	Nasal bone
13	Lacrimal sac (upper extremity)
14	Upper lacrimal canaliculus
15	Upper lacrimal punctum with black bristle in papilla
16	Lower lacrimal canaliculus
17	Lower lacrimal punctum with black bristle in papilla
18	Orbicularis oculi (palpebral part)
19	Aponeurosis of levator palpebrae superioris
20	Orbital fat pad
21	Nasolacrimal duct
22	Infra-orbital nerve in infra-orbital foramen
23	Lacrimal artery and nerve
24	Orbital part ⎤ of lacrimal
25	Palpebral part ⎦ gland
26	Aponeurosis of levator palpebrae superioris

The lacrimal gland:
➤ Tucks into the upper (roof), and outer (lateral) corner of the bony orbit.
➤ Has an orbital (upper) and palpebral (lower) part.
➤ Through a dozen or so ducts constantly supplies a watery secretion to the surface of the eyeball.
➤ The fluid drains across the eyeball to the upper and lower lacrimal punctum situated in the inner corner of the upper and lower eyelids, into the canaliculus, the lacrimal sac and nasolacrimal duct where it descends, finally flowing out into the inferior meatus.

A Left auricle – *from the left*

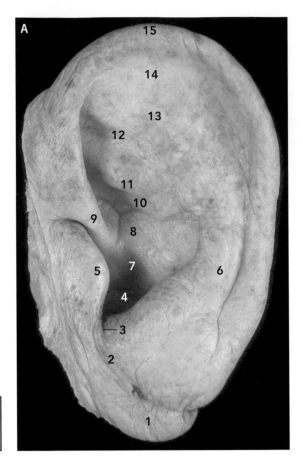

1   Lobule
2   Antitragus
3   Intertragic notch
4   External acoustic meatus
5   Tragus
6   Antihelix
7   Cavum conchae
8   Concha
9   Crus of helix
10 Cymba conchae
11 Lower crus of antihelix
12 Triangular fossa
13 Upper crus of antihelix
14 Scaphoid fossa
15 Helix

B Left auricular cartilage (pinna) – *from the left*

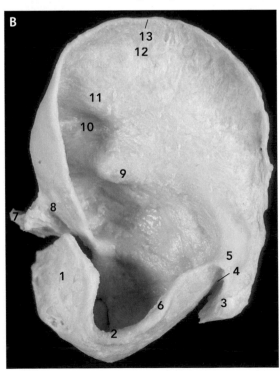

1   Cartilage of external acoustic meatus
2   Intratragic notch
3   Tail of helix
4   Antitragohelicine meatus
5   Antihelix
6   Antitragus
7   Spine of helix
8   Crus of helix
9   Lower crus of antihelix
10 Triangular fossa
11 Upper crus of antihelix
12 Scaphoid fossa
13 Helix

Adult skull without the mandible, lower lateral surface – *from the left and slightly below*

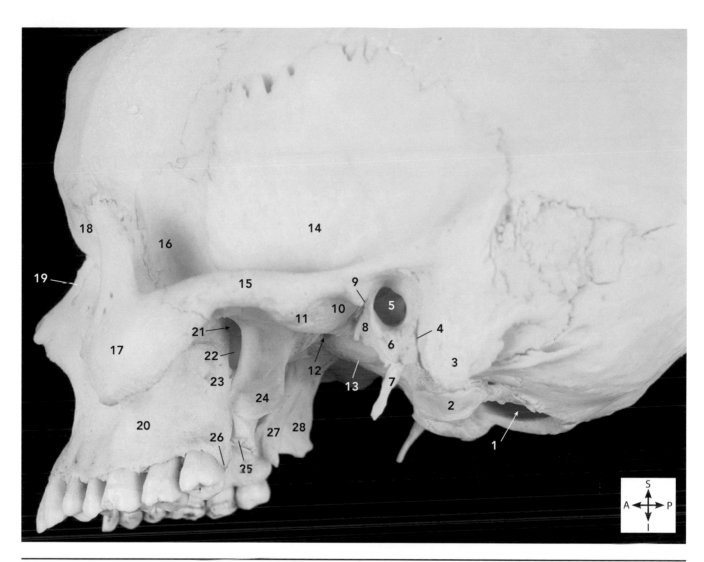

1	Foramen magnum	16	Greater wing of sphenoid
2	Occipital condyle	17	Zygomatic bone
3	Mastoid process	18	Frontal bone
4	Tympanomastoid fissure	19	Nasal bone
5	External acoustic meatus	20	Maxilla
6	Sheath of styloid process	21	Sphenopalatine foramen
7	Styloid process	22	Pterygomaxillary fissure
8	Tympanic part of temporal bone	23	Infratemporal surface of maxilla
9	Squamotympanic fissure	24	Lateral pterygoid plate
10	Mandibular fossa	25	Pyramidal process of palatine bone
11	Articular tubercle	26	Tuberosity of maxilla
12	Foramen ovale	27	Right medial ⎤ pterygoid plate
13	Pharyngeal tubercle	28	Right lateral ⎦
14	Squamous part ⎤ of temporal		
15	Zygomatic process ⎦ bone		

Left inner ear exposed through the tegmen tympani of the temporal bone in the floor of the middle cranial fossa – *from above*

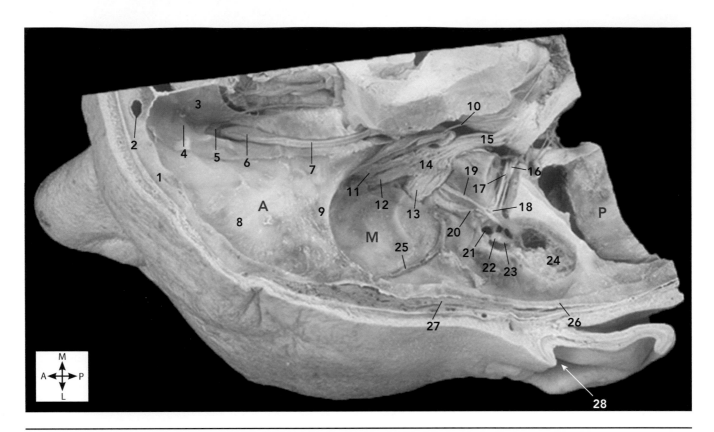

A	Anterior		9	Lesser wing of sphenoid
M	Middle	cranial fossa	10	Trochlear nerve (IV)
P	Posterior		11	Ophthalmic nerve (V¹)

A Anterior
M Middle ⎤ cranial fossa
P Posterior ⎦

1 Frontal bone
2 Frontal sinus
3 Falx cerebri
4 Crista galli of ethmoid bone
5 Cribriform plate of ethmoid bone
6 Olfactory bulb
7 Olfactory tract
8 Orbital part of frontal bone

9 Lesser wing of sphenoid
10 Trochlear nerve (IV)
11 Ophthalmic nerve (V^1)
12 Maxillary nerve (V^2)
13 Mandibular nerve (V^3)
14 Trigeminal ganglion
15 Trigeminal nerve (V)
16 Vestibulocochlear nerve ⎤ in internal
   (VIII) and artery   ⎥ acoustic meatus
17 Facial nerve (VII)   ⎦
18 Geniculate ganglion
19 Greater ⎤ petrosal nerve
20 Lesser ⎦

21 Cavity of middle ear
22 Malleus
23 Incus
24 Mastoid air cells
25 Frontal branch of middle meningeal artery
26 Squamous part of temporal bone
27 Temporalis
28 External acoustic meatus

Coronal section through the left ear – *from behind*

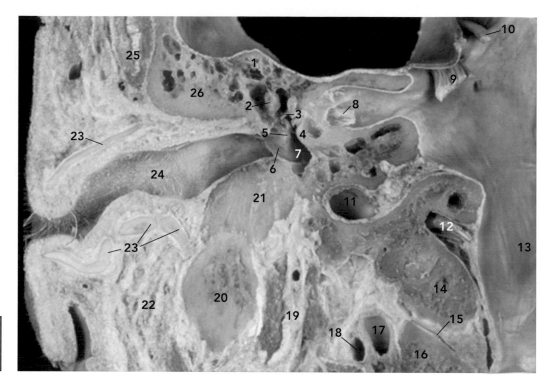

1 Tegmen tympani	10 Oculomotor nerve (IV)	18 Vertebral vein
2 Head of malleus	11 Internal jugular vein	19 Styloid process
3 Tendon of tensor tympani	12 Glossopharyngeal (IX), vagus (X) and accessory nerve (XI) in jugular foramen	20 Head of mandible (posterior part)
4 Promontory of middle ear		21 Tympanic part of temporal bone
5 Handle of malleus	13 Dura mater covering clivus	22 Parotid gland
6 Tympanic membrane	14 Occipital condyle	23 Auricular cartilage
7 Cavity of middle ear	15 Atlanto-occipital joint	24 External acoustic meatus
8 Facial (VII) and vestibulocochlear nerve (VIII) in internal acoustic meatus	16 Lateral mass of atlas (first [CI] cervical vertebra)	25 Temporalis
	17 Vertebral artery	26 Temporal bone
9 Trigeminal nerve (V)		

Coronal section through the left ear – *from the front*

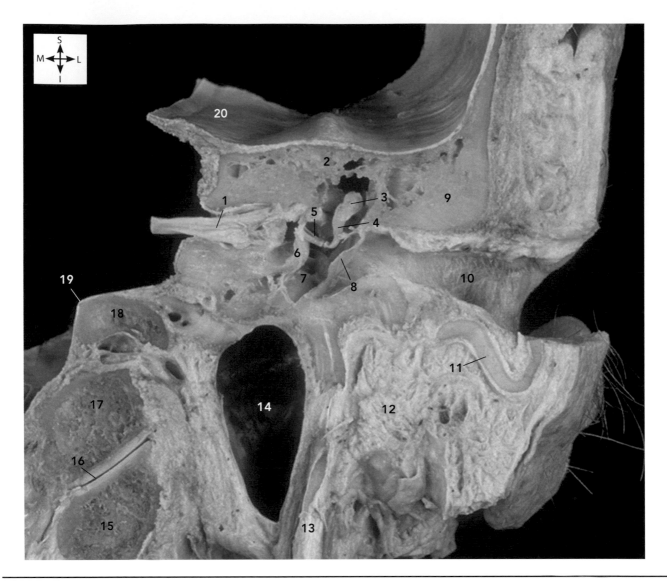

1	Facial (VII) and vestibulocochlear nerve (VIII) in internal acoustic meatus	7 Cavity of middle ear
2	Tegmen tympani	8 Tympanic membrane
3	Head of malleus	9 Temporal bone
4	Long limb of incus	10 External acoustic meatus
5	Stapes	11 Auricular cartilage
6	Promontory of middle ear	12 Parotid gland
		13 Styloid process
		14 Internal jugular vein
		15 Atlas (first [CI] cervical vertebra)
		16 Atlanto-occipital joint
		17 Occipital condyle
		18 Basilar part of occipital bone
		19 Margin of foramen magnum
		20 Dura mater lining floor of middle cranial fossa

The external ear:

➤ Comprises of the auricle (the pinna) and the external acoustic meatus, at the medial end of which is situated the thin transparent tympanic membrane.

➤ The tympanic membrane forms a barrier which seperates the external ear from the middle ear (tympanic cavity).

The middle ear – the tympanic cavity:

➤ Is an irregular space within the temporal bone lined with mucous membrane.

➤ It contains the three auditory ossicles (the malleus, incus and stapes).

➤ Is filled with air which communicates anteriorly with the nasopharynx via the auditory tube.

PART II

Vertebral Column, Spinal Cord, Skeleton and Trunk

Adult skeleton of the vertebral column – *from the left*

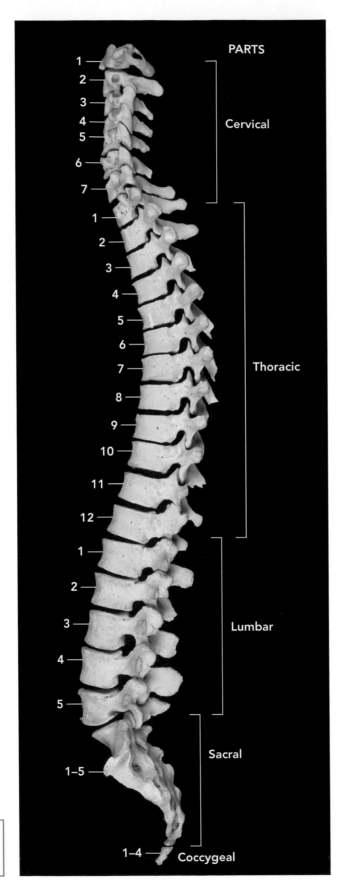

PARTS

Cervical

Thoracic

Lumbar

Sacral

Coccygeal

Cervical vertebra

1 First (CI) – atlas
2 Second (CII) – axis
3 Third (CIII)
4 Fourth (CIV)
5 Fifth (CV)
6 Sixth (CVI)
7 Seventh (CVII) – vertebra prominens

Thoracic vertebra

1 First (TI)
2 Second (TII)
3 Third (TIII)
4 Fourth (TIV)
5 Fifth (TV)
6 Sixth (TVI)
7 Seventh (TVII)
8 Eighth (TVIII)
9 Ninth (TIX)
10 Tenth (TX)
11 Eleventh (TXI)
12 Twelfth (TXII)

Lumbar vertebra

1 First (LI)
2 Second (LII)
3 Third (LIII)
4 Fourth (LIV)
5 Fifth (LV)

Sacrum 1–5

Normally formed from the fusion of five sacral vertebra (sacral vertebrae I–V).

Coccyx 1–4

Normally formed by fusion of four rudimentary vertebra (but variable three to five) (coccygeal vertebrae I–IV).

Adult skeleton, with long bones of the left upper and lower limb removed – *from the left*

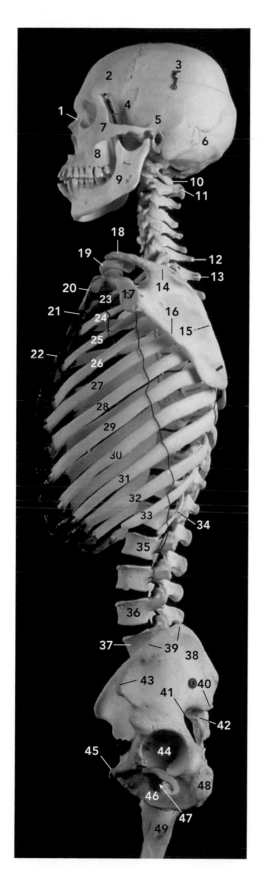

1 Nasal bone
2 Frontal bone
3 Parietal bone
4 Sphenoid
5 Temporal bone
6 Occipital bone
7 Zygomatic bone
8 Maxilla
9 Mandible
10 First (CI) cervical vertebra – atlas
11 Second (CII) cervical vertebra – axis
12 Seventh (CVII) cervical vertebra – vertebra prominens
13 First (TI) thoracic vertebra
14 Spine ⎤
15 Medial border ⎥
16 Lateral border ⎬ of scapula
17 Glenoid cavity ⎥
18 Acromion ⎦
19 Acromial end of clavicle
20 Manubrium of sternum
21 Manubriosternal joint
22 Body of sternum
23 First (I) ⎤
24 Second (II) ⎥
25 Third (III) ⎥
26 Fourth (IV) ⎥
27 Fifth (V) ⎥
28 Sixth (VI) ⎥
29 Seventh (VII) ⎬ rib
30 Eighth (VIII) ⎥
31 Ninth (IX) ⎥
32 Tenth (X) ⎥
33 Eleventh (XI) ⎥
34 Twelfth (XII) ⎦
35 Second (LII) ⎤
36 Fourth (LIV) ⎬ lumbar vertebra
37 Fifth (LV) ⎦
38 Hip bone
39 Iliac crest
40 Posterior inferior iliac spine
41 Greater sciatic notch
42 Sacrum
43 Anterior superior iliac spine
44 Acetabulum
45 Pubic tubercle
46 Body of pubis
47 Obturator foramen
48 Ischial tuberosity
49 Shaft of right femur

A   **Adult first (CI) cervical vertebra – atlas –** *from above*

B   **Adult second (CII) cervical vertebra – axis –** *from above*

C   **Adult fifth (CV) cervical vertebra –** *from above*

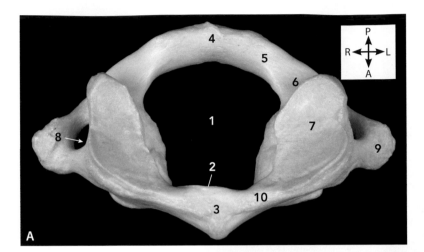

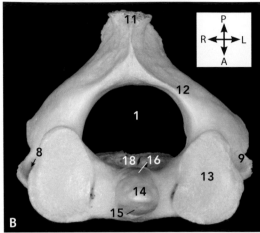

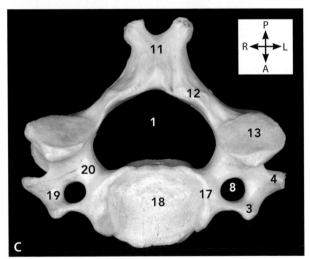

1 Vertebral foramen	8 Foramen transversarium	15 Anterior ⎤ articular surface
2 Facet for dens of axis	9 Transverse process	16 Posterior ⎦ of dens
3 Anterior ⎤ tubercle	10 Anterior arch	17 Uncus (posterolateral lip) of body
4 Posterior ⎦	11 Bifid spinous process	18 Body
5 Posterior arch	12 Lamina	19 Groove for spinal nerve (ventral
6 Groove for vertebral artery	13 Superior articular process	ramus)
7 Lateral mass with superior articular facet	14 Apex of dens	20 Pedicle

The foramen transversarium:
➤ Is present in the transverse processes of all seven cervical vertebrae, a feature that distinguishes them from the rest of the vertebrae forming the vertebral column.
➤ The foramen accommodates the vertebral artery, which enters the sixth vertebra, ascends through the remaining five to loop into the foramen magnum.

The typical cervical vertebrae:
➤ Are deemed the third to the sixth; the first (CI) (atlas), second (CII) (axis) and seventh (CVII) (vertebra prominens) differ, having certain distinct features.

A   Adult first (TI) thoracic vertebra – *from above*

B   Adult fourth (LIV) lumbar vertebra – *from above*

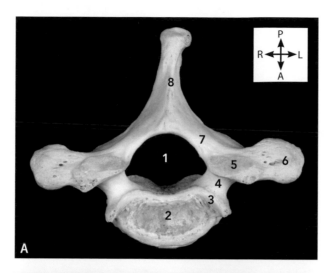

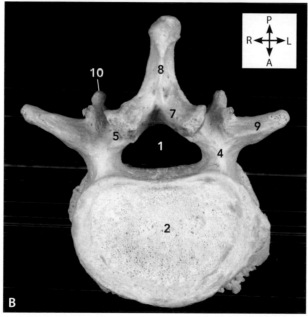

1 Vertebral foramen	5 Superior articular process	8 Spinous process
2 Body	6 Transverse process with costal	9 Transverse process
3 Posterolateral lip (uncus)	facet	10 Mamillary process
4 Pedicle	7 Lamina	

The typical thoracic vertebrae:
➤ Are the second to the ninth having characteristic features of upper and lower articular facets on the sides of their bodies, which join the heads of the ribs, and an articular facet on the front of each transverse process, which joins a rib tubercle.
➤ They also have, a round vertebral foramen, spinous process that points downwards and backwards, and superior articular processes that are vertical, flat and face backwards and laterally.

The lumbar vertebrae:
➤ Have large sized bodies, no costal facets on their bodies and transverse processes, and a distinct triangular-shaped vertebral foramen.

Skull and vertebral column, with posterior half of the cranium removed and vertebral canal opened to expose the brain and spinal cord *in situ* – *from behind*

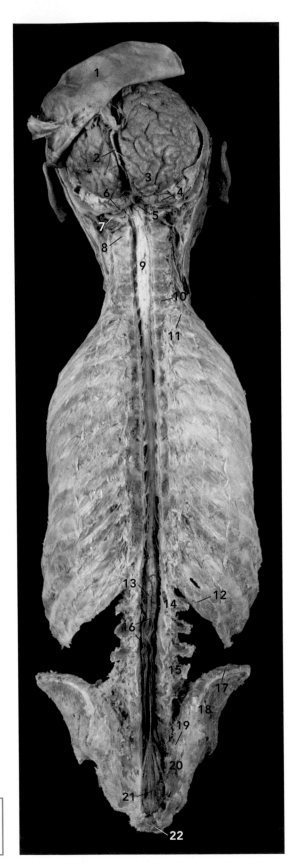

1 Dura mater (reflected superiorly)
2 Falx cerebri
3 Occipital pole of the right cerebral hemisphere
4 Right cerebellar hemisphere
5 Medulla oblongata
6 Margin of foramen magnum
7 First (CI) cervical vertebra – atlas
8 Second (CII) cervical vertebra – axis
9 Spinal medulla (spinal cord)
10 Seventh (CVII) cervical vertebra – vertebra prominens
11 First rib (I)
12 Eleventh rib (XI)
13 Conus medularis of spinal cord
14 First (LI) ⎤
15 Fourth (LIV) ⎦ lumbar vertebra
16 Cauda equina
17 Iliac crest
18 Hip bone
19 Sacroiliac joint
20 Sacrum
21 Filum terminale
22 Coccyx

The medulla oblongata:
➤ Is the lowest part of the brainstem and at the level of the foramen magnum becomes continuous with the spinal medulla (spinal cord).

The spinal medulla (spinal cord):
➤ Normally ends at the level of the first (LI) lumbar vertebra where it forms the conus medularis; below this point it becomes the cauda equina (*the horse's tail*), which is formed from dorsal and ventral roots of the lumbar, sacral and coccygeal nerves.

The vertebral artery:
➤ Enters the foramen transversarium of the sixth (CVI) cervical vertebra.

The vertebral vein:
➤ Emerges from the foramen transversarium of the seventh (CVII) cervical vertebra and occasionally may be accompanied by a much smaller vein that passes from the sixth (CVI) cervical vertebra.

Skull and cervical part of the vertebral column, with the posterior part of the cranium removed, vertebral canal exposed and spinal cord partially removed – *from behind*

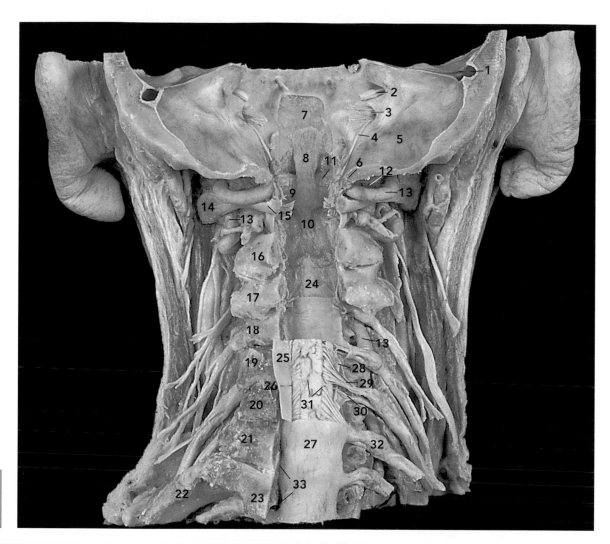

1 Transverse sinus
2 Facial nerve (VII), vestibulocochlear nerve (VIII), labyrinthine artery, in internal acoustic meatus
3 Glossopharyngeal nerve (IX), vagus nerve (X) and accessory nerves (XI), in jugular foramen
4 Spinal root of accessory nerve (XI)
5 Dura mater lining floor of posterior cranial fossa
6 Margin of foramen magnum
7 Basilar part of occipital bone
8 Superior longitudinal band of cruciform ligament

9 Transverse ligament of atlas
10 Inferior longitudinal band of cruciform ligament
11 Alar ligament
12 Atlanto-occipital joint
13 Vertebral artery
14 Transverse process ⎤ of atlas – first
15 Posterior arch ⎦ (CI) cervical vertebra
16 Second (CII) cervical vertebra – axis
17 Third (CIII) ⎤
18 Fourth (CIV) ⎤ cervical vertebra
19 Fifth (CV) ⎤
20 Sixth (CVI) ⎦

21 Seventh (CVII) cervical vertebra – vertebra prominens
22 First (I) rib
23 First (TI) thoracic vertebra
24 Posterior longitudinal ligament
25 Arachnoid and dura mater (reflected)
26 Subarachnoid space
27 Dura mater
28 Denticulate ligament
29 Dorsal ⎤ rootlets of
30 Ventral ⎦ spinal nerve
31 Posterior spinal arteries
32 Dural sheath over dorsal root ganglion
33 Extradural space

Adult skeleton of the trunk – *from the front*

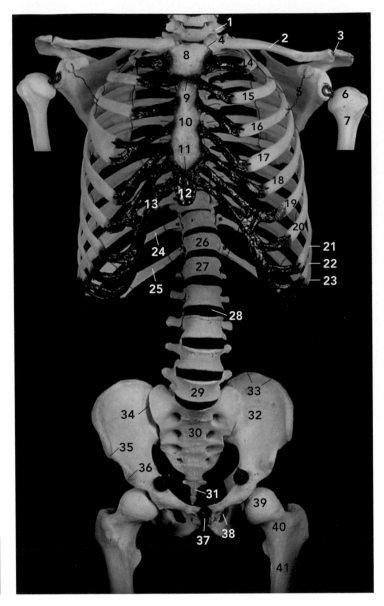

1	Seventh (CVII) cervical vertebra – vertebra prominens	14	First (I)	28	Intervertebral disc (synthetic representation)
2	Body of clavicle	15	Second (II)	29	Fifth (LV) lumbar vertebra
3	Acromioclavicular joint	16	Third (III)	30	Sacrum
4	Sternoclavicular joint	17	Fourth (IV)	31	Coccyx
5	Scapula	18	Fifth (V)	32	Hip bone
6	Head ⎤ of humerus	19	Sixth (VI)	33	Iliac crest
7	Surgical neck ⎦	20	Seventh (VII) rib	34	Sacro-iliac joint
8	Manubrium of sternum	21	Eighth (VIII)	35	Anterior superior ⎤ iliac spine
9	Manubriosternal joint	22	Ninth (IX)	36	Anterior inferior ⎦
10	Body of sternum	23	Tenth (X)	37	Pubic symphysis
11	Xiphisternal joint	24	Eleventh (XI)	38	Obturator foramen
12	Xiphoid process	25	Twelfth (XII)	39	Head ⎤
13	Seventh costal cartilage	26	Twelfth (TXII) thoracic vertebra	40	Neck ⎥ of femur
		27	First (LI) lumbar vertebra	41	Shaft ⎦

Anterior muscles of the trunk – *from the front*

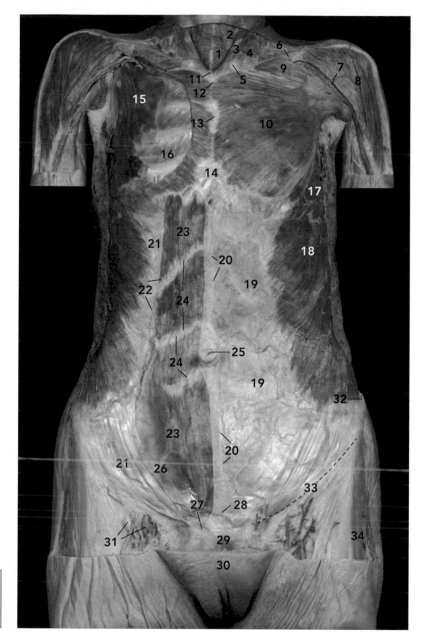

1 Sternohyoid	12 Manubrium ⎤ of sternum	24 Tedinous intersection of rectus abdominis
2 Sternothyroid	13 Body ⎦	
3 Sternal ⎤ head of sterno-	14 Xiphoid process	25 Umbilicus
4 Clavicular ⎦ cleidomastoid	15 Pectoralis minor	26 Posterior layer of internal oblique aponeurosis
5 Capsule of sternoclavicular joint	16 Internal intercostal	
	17 Serratus anterior	27 Pubic tubercle
6 Body of clavicle	18 External oblique	28 Pyrymidalis
7 Cephalic vein in deltopectoral groove	19 Rectus sheath	29 Pubic symphysis
	20 Linea alba	30 Mons pubis
8 Deltoid	21 External oblique aponeurosis	31 Superficial inguinal lymph nodes
9 Clavicular ⎤ part of	22 Linea semilunaris	32 Iliac crest
10 Sternocostal ⎦ pectoralis major	23 Rectus abdominis	33 Inguinal ligament
11 Suprasternal notch		34 Tensor fascia latae

Adult skeleton of the trunk – *from behind*

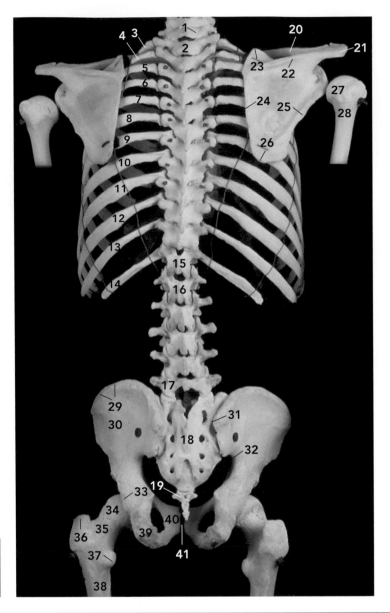

1	Seventh (CVII) cervical vertebra – vertebra prominens	
2	First (TI) thoracic vertebra	
3	First (I)	
4	Second (II)	
5	Third (III)	
6	Fourth (IV)	
7	Fifth (V)	
8	Sixth (VI)	rib
9	Seventh (VII)	
10	Eighth (VIII)	
11	Ninth IX)	
12	Tenth (X)	
13	Eleventh (XI)	
14	Twelfth (XII)	
15	Twelfth (TXII) thoracic vertebra	
16	First (LI)	lumbar vertebra
17	Fifth (LV)	
18	Sacrum	
19	Coccyx	
20	Body of clavicle	
21	Acromion	
22	Spine	
23	Superior angle	of scapula
24	Medial border	
25	Later border	
26	Inferior angle	
27	Head	of humerus
28	Surgical neck	
29	Iliac crest	
30	Hip bone	
31	Sacroiliac joint	
32	Greater sciatic notch	
33	Rim of acetabulum	
34	Head	
35	Neck	
36	Greater trochanter	of femur
37	Lesser trochanter	
38	Shaft	
39	Ischium	
40	Pubis	
41	Pubic symphysis	

Posterior muscles of the trunk – *from behind*

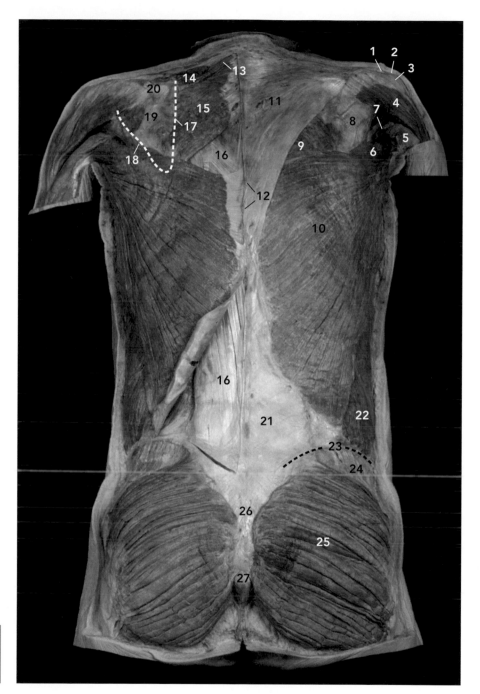

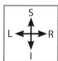

1	Acromial end of clavicle	11	Trapezius
2	Acromioclavicular joint (position of)	12	Spinous processes of cervical vertebrae
3	Acromion of scapula	13	Rhomboid minor
4	Deltoid	14	Levator scapulae
5	Long head of triceps	15	Rhomboid major
6	Teres major	16	Erector spinae
7	Teres minor	17	Medial border (position of
8	Infraspinatus	18	Lateral border scapula)
9	Triangle of auscultation	19	Fascia overlying infraspinatus
10	Latissimus dorsi		

20 Spine of scapula (position of)
21 Thoracolumbar fascia overlying erector spinae
22 External oblique
23 Iliac crest
24 Gluteus medius
25 Gluteus maximus
26 Sacrum
27 Coccyx

PART III

Upper Limb

Adult bones of the left upper limb – *A from the front; B from behind*

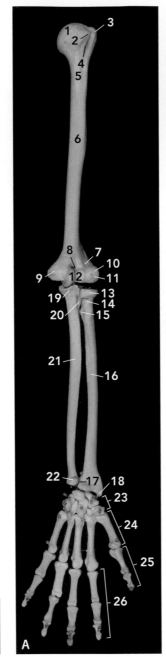

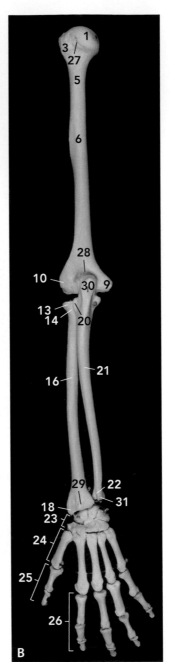

1	Head of humerus	
2	Lesser ⎫ tubercle	
3	Greater ⎭	
4	Interterbercular sulcus	
5	Surgical neck	
6	Shaft of humerus	
7	Radial fossa	
8	Coronoid fossa	
9	Medial ⎫ epicondyle	
10	Lateral ⎭	
11	Capitulum	
12	Trochlea	
13	Head ⎫ of radius	
14	Neck ⎭	
15	Tuberosity	
16	Shaft of radius	
17	Ulnar notch	
18	Styloid process	
19	Coronoid process ⎫	
20	Supinator crest ⎪	
21	Shaft ⎬ of ulna	
22	Head ⎭	
23	Eight carpal bones of hand	
24	Five (I–V) metacarpal bones of hand	
25	Two phalanges of thumb	
26	Twelve phalanges of fingers	
27	Anatomical neck of humerus	
28	Olecranon fossa	
29	Dorsal tubercle of radius	
30	Olecranon ⎫ of ulna	
31	Styloid process ⎭	

Coronal section through the left shoulder joint – *from the front*

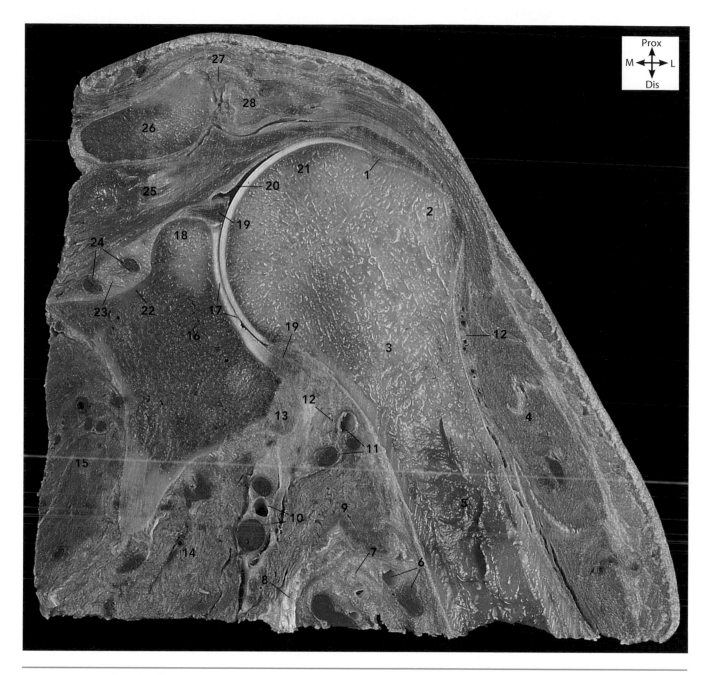

1	Anatomical neck ⎤	11	Posterior circumflex artery and vein
2	Greater tubercle ⎟ of humerus	12	Axillary nerve
3	Surgical neck ⎦	13	Long head of triceps
4	Deltoid	14	Teres minor
5	Shaft of humerus	15	Subscapularis
6	Brachial artery and vein	16	Head ⎤
7	Nerves of brachial plexus	17	Glenoid fossa ⎟ of scapula
8	Tendon of teres major	18	Coracoid process ⎦
9	Latissimus dorsi	19	Glenoid labrum
10	Medial circumflex scapular artery and vein	20	Cavity of shoulder joint

21	Head of humerus
22	Neck of scapula
23	Suprascapular nerve
24	Suprascapular vessels
25	Supraspinatus
26	Acromial end of clavicle
27	Acromioclavicular joint
28	Acromion of scapula

Superficial structures of the left anterior thoracic wall and shoulder –
from the front and slightly right

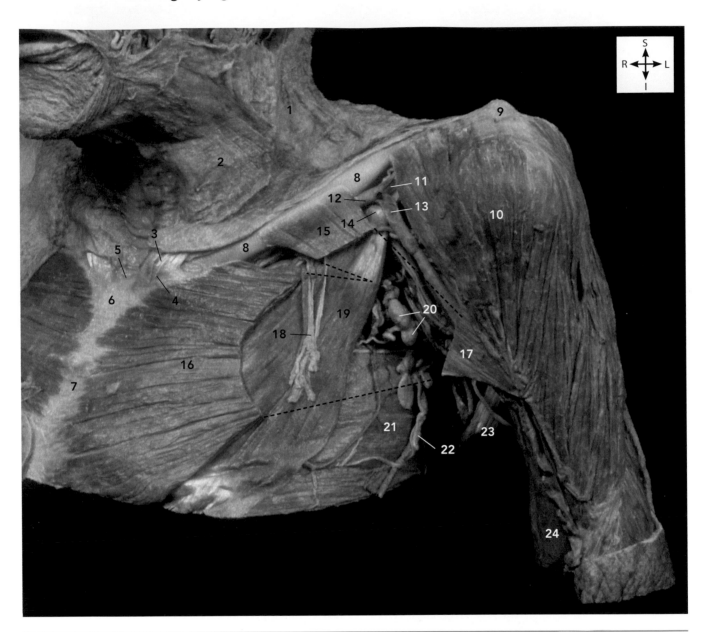

1	Investing layer of lateral cervical fascia	
2	Platysma	
3	Sternal head of sternocleidomastoid	
4	Sternoclavicular joint	
5	Suprasternal notch	
6	Manubrium ⎤ of sternum	
7	Body ⎦	
8	Body of clavicle	
9	Acromioclavicular joint	
10	Deltoid	
11	Axillary vein	
12	Subclavian vein	
13	Cephalic vein in deltopectoral triangle	
14	Position of coracoid process of scapula	
15	Clavicular ⎤ part of pectoralis major	
16	Sternocostal ⎦	
17	Common origin of pectoralis major	
18	Thoraco-acromial vessels and lateral pectoral nerve	
19	Pectoralis minor	
20	Axillary lymph nodes (cluster)	
21	Serratus anterior	
22	Thoracodorsal artery and long thoracic nerve	
23	Latissimus dorsi	
24	Biceps	

Structures of the left deep lateral neck, brachial plexus, axilla, shoulder and upper arm – *from the front*

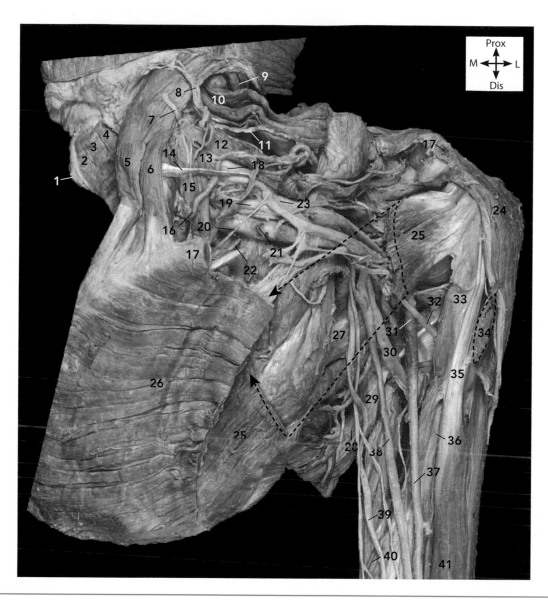

1	Laryngeal prominence of thyroid cartilage	15	Scalenus anterior	29	Latissimus dorsi
2	Sternohyoid	16	Thyrocervical trunk	30	Axillary vein
3	Superior belly of omohyoid	17	Body of clavicle	31	Axillary artery
4	Thyrohyoid	18	Upper trunk of brachial plexus	32	Musculocutaneous nerve
5	Sternal ⎤ head of	19	Subclavian artery	33	Short head of biceps fused with coracobrachialis
6	Clavicular ⎦ sternocleidomastoid	20	Accessory phrenic nerve	34	Pectoralis major (common origin)
7	Transverse cervical nerve	21	Subclavian vein	35	Long head of biceps
8	Great auricular nerve	22	Inferior thoracic artery	36	Coracobrachialis
9	Splenius capitis	23	Brachial plexus	37	Brachial artery
10	Levator scapulae	24	Deltoid	38	Median nerve
11	Accessory nerve	25	Pectoralis minor	39	Ulnar nerve
12	Scalenus medius	26	Pectoralis major	40	Triceps
13	Superficial cervical artery	27	Subscapularis	41	Biceps
14	Inferior belly of omohyoid	28	Teres major		

Left brachial plexus and axilla I – *from the front*

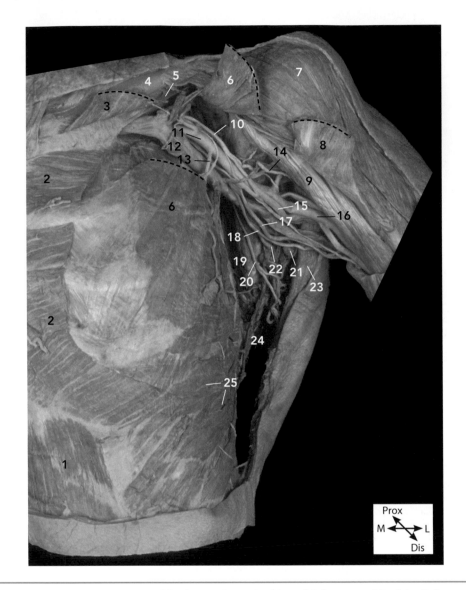

1	Rectus abdominis	10	Lateral cord of brachial plexus	18	Medial cutaneous nerve of arm
2	Sternocostal ⎤ part of pectoralis	11	Axillary artery	19	Subscapularis
3	Clavicular ⎦ major	12	Axillary vein	20	Thoracodorsal nerve
4	Body of clavicle	13	Lateral thoracic artery	21	Axillary lymph node
5	Subclavius	14	Musculocutaneous nerve	22	Thoracodorsal artery
6	Pectoralis minor	15	Median nerve	23	Latissimus dorsi
7	Deltoid	16	Brachial artery	24	Teres major
8	Pectoralis major (common origin)	17	Ulnar nerve	25	Serratus anterior
9	Coracobrachialis and short head of biceps				

The cords of the brachial plexus – located around the axillary artery are:

➤ **Lateral cord** – major branches: the musculocutaneous nerve, lateral root of the median nerve and the lateral pectoral nerve.

➤ **Medial cord** – major branches: the ulnar nerve, medial root of the median nerve, the medial pectoral nerve and the medial cutaneous nerves of the arm and forearm.

➤ **Posterior cord** – major branches: the radial nerve, axillary nerve, subscapular nerves and thoracodorsal nerve.

Left brachial plexus and axilla II – *from the front*

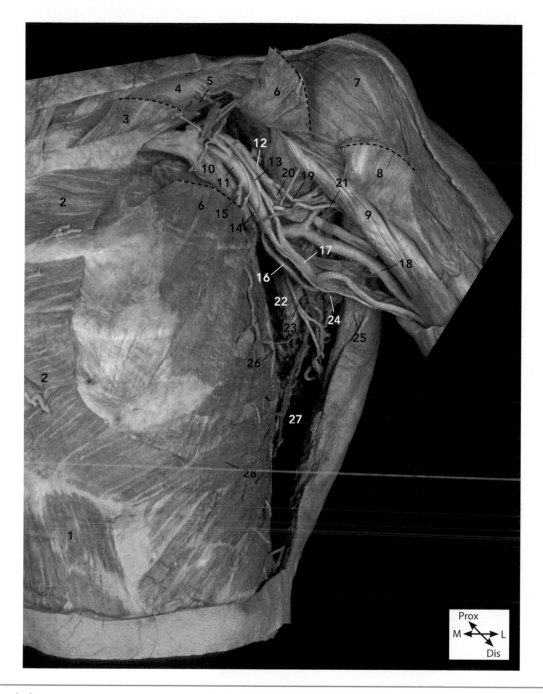

1	Rectus abdominis	10	Axillary vein
2	Sternocostal ⎤ part of pectoralis	11	Axillary artery
3	Clavicular ⎦ major	12	Posterior cord ⎤
4	Body of clavicle	13	Lateral cord ⎥ of brachial plexus
5	Subclavius	14	Medial cord ⎦
6	Pectoralis minor	15	Lateral thoracic artery
7	Deltoid	16	Ulnar ⎤ nerve
8	Pectoralis major (common origin)	17	Median ⎦
9	Coracobrachialis and short head of biceps	18	Brachial artery
		19	Axillary ⎤ nerve
		20	Radial ⎦

21	Musculocutaneous nerve
22	Subscapularis
23	Thoracodorsal nerve
24	Axillary lymph node
25	Latissimus dorsi
26	Long thoracic nerve
27	Teres major
28	Serratus anterior

Coronal section through the left elbow joint – *from the front*

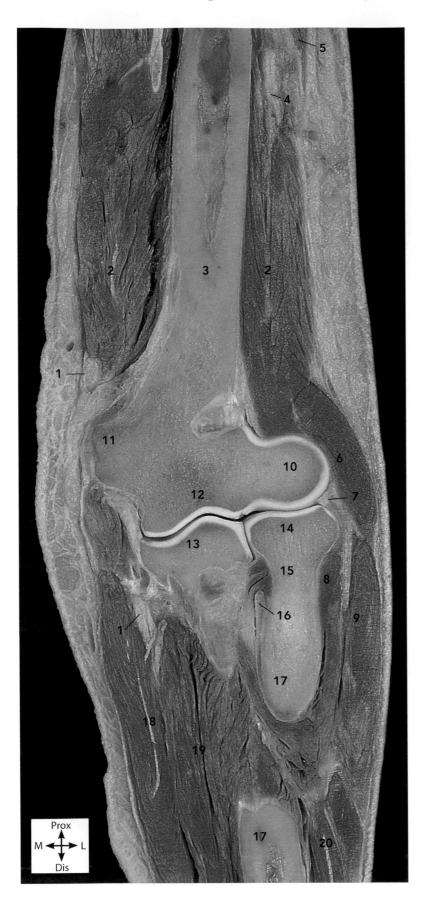

1   Ulnar nerve
2   Medial head of triceps
3   Shaft of humerus
4   Radial nerve
5   Lateral head of triceps
6   Brachioradialis
7   Annular ligament
8   Supinator
9   Extensor carpi radialis longus
10 Capitulum
11 Medial epicondyle ⎤ of humerus
12 Trochlea   ⎦
13 Coronoid process of ulna
14 Head ⎤ of radius
15 Neck ⎦
16 Tendon of biceps
17 Shaft of radius
18 Flexor carpi ulnaris
19 Flexor digitorum profundus
20 Extensor carpi radialis brevis

The elbow joint:
➤ Is formed between the lower end of
   the humerus and upper ends of the
   ulna and radius.
➤ The trochlea of the humerus articulates
   with the trochlear notch of the ulna,
   and the capitulum of the humerus
   articulates with the upper surface of
   the head of the radius.
➤ The head of the radius and the ulna
   also articulate with one another to
   form the proximal radio-ulnar joint
   where they are held together by the
   annular ligament.

Adult bones of the left elbow joint – *A from the front; B from behind*

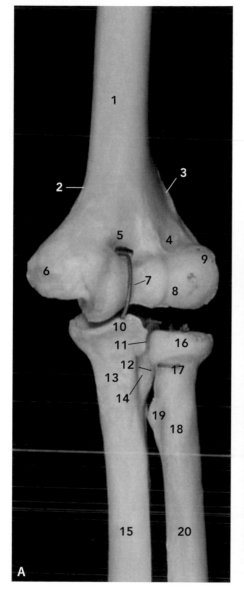

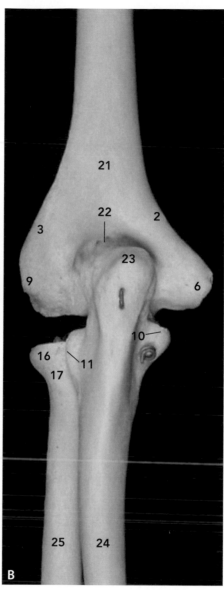

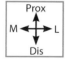

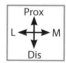

1	Anterior surface	16	Head
2	Medial supracondylar ridge	17	Neck
3	Lateral supracondylar ridge	18	Tuberosity
4	Radial fossa	19	Rough area for pronator teres
5	Coronoid fossa	20	Anterior surface
6	Medial epicondyle	21	Posterior surface
7	Trochlea	22	Olecranon fossa
8	Capitulum	23	Olecranon
9	Lateral epicondyle	24	Posterior surface
10	Coronoid process	25	Posterior surface of radius
11	Radial notch		
12	Supinator crest		
13	Tuberosity		
14	Supinator surface		
15	Anterior surface		

1–9 of humerus

18–20 of radius

21–22 of humerus

23–24 of ulna

10–15 of ulna

Structures of the left anterior shoulder, upper arm and forearm –
from the front

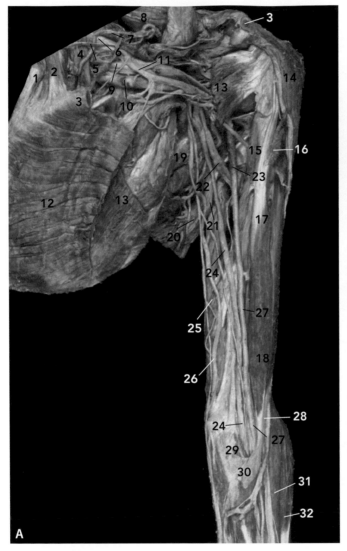

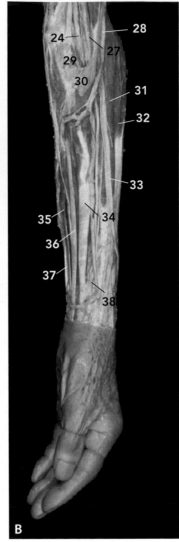

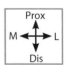

A

B

1	Sternal ⎤ of	15	Short head of	26	Ulnar nerve
2	Clavicular head ⎦ sternocleidomastoid		biceps fused with	27	Brachial artery
3	Clavicle		coracobrachialis	28	Tendon of biceps
4	Scalenus anterior	16	Pectoralis major	29	Pronator teres
5	Inferior belly of omohyoid		(common origin)	30	Bicipital aponeurosis
6	Upper trunk of brachial plexus	17	Long head of biceps	31	Brachioradialis
7	Scalenus medius	18	Biceps	32	Extensor carpi radialis longus
8	Levator scapulae	19	Subscapularis	33	Cephalic vein
9	Subclavian artery	20	Teres major	34	Flexor carpi radialis
10	Subclavian vein	21	Latissimus dorsi	35	Palmaris longus
11	Brachial plexus	22	Axillary vein	36	Flexor digitorum superficialis
12	Pectoralis major	23	Axillary artery	37	Flexor carpi ulnaris
13	Pectoralis minor	24	Median nerve	38	Radial artery
14	Deltoid	25	Triceps		

Structures of the left posterior upper arm and forearm – *from behind*

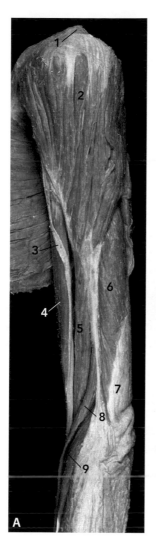
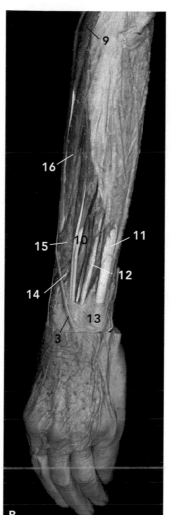

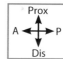

Prox

A ◄► P

Dis

A

B

Prox

A ◄► P

Dis

1	Acromioclavicular joint	7	Tendon of triceps	13	Extensor retinaculum
2	Deltoid	8	Brachioradialis	14	Extensor pollicis brevis
3	Cephalic vein	9	Extensor carpi radialis longus	15	Abductor pollicis longus
4	Biceps	10	Extensor digitorum	16	Extensor carpi radialis brevis
5	Coracobrachialis	11	Extensor carpi ulnaris		
6	Triceps	12	Extensor digiti minimi		

The cubital fossa:
➤ Is a triangular-shaped region at the front of the elbow the boundaries of which are:
  ➤ **Medially** – pronator teres.
  ➤ **Laterally** – brachioradialis.
  ➤ **Above** – a line between the humeral epicondyles.
  ➤ **Floor** – formed by brachialis and supinator.

The brachial artery:
➤ At the cubital fossa, may be palpated with the elbow straight and pressing on the medial side of the biceps tendon.

The median nerve:
➤ Lies just medial to the brachial artery.

Superficial structures of the left forearm and palm of hand – *from the front*

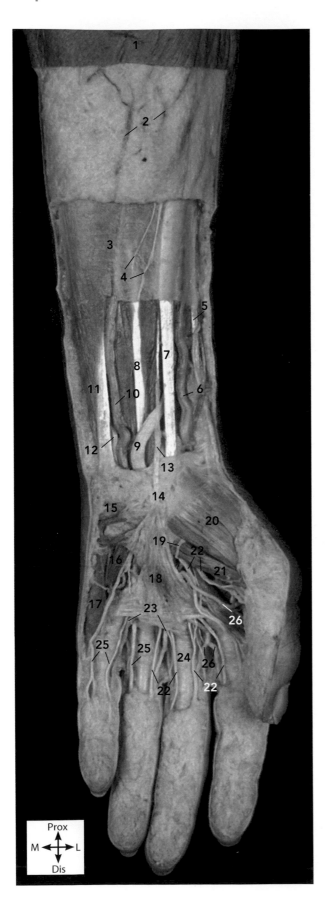

1   Skin of forearm
2   Superficial veins within subcutaneous tissue
3   Deep fascia of forearm
4   Branches of medial cutaneous nerve of forearm
5   Brachioradialis
6   Radial artery
7   Flexor carpi radialis
8   Flexor digitorum superficialis
9   Median nerve
10 Ulnar artery
11 Flexor carpi ulnaris
12 Ulnar nerve
13 Palmaris longus
14 Flexor retinaculum
15 Palmaris brevis
16 Flexor digitorum minimi brevis
17 Abductor digiti minimi
18 Central part of palmar aponeurosis
19 Recurrent branch of median nerve
20 Abductor policis brevis
21 Flexor policis brevis
22 Digital branches of median nerve
23 Common palmar digital arteries
24 Fibrous sheath of middle finger
25 Digital branches of ulnar nerve
26 Proper palmar digital artery

The radial artery pulse:
➤ Is felt by pressing the artery against the lower end of the radius, on the radial (lateral) side of the tendon of flexor carpi radialis.

The ulnar artery pulse:
➤ Is less easy to palpate but usually can be felt on the radial side of the tendon of flexor carpi ulnaris, just before its attachment to the pisiform bone.

Superficial structures of the left distal forearm and dorsum of hand – *from behind*

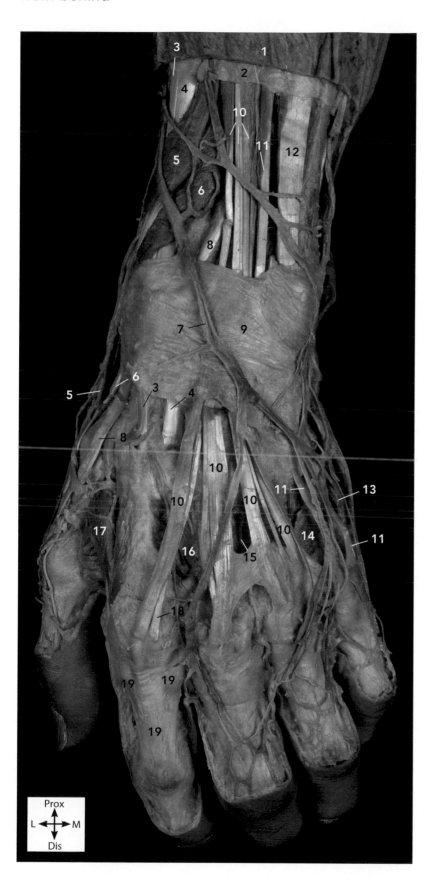

1 Skin of forearm
2 Deep fascia of forearm
3 Extensor carpi radialis longus
4 Extensor carpi radialis brevis
5 Abductor pollicis longus
6 Extensor pollicis brevis
7 Cephalic vein
8 Extensor pollicis longus
9 Extensor retinaculum
10 Extensor digitorum
11 Extensor digiti minimi
12 Extensor carpi ulnaris
13 Abductor digiti minimi
14 Fourth ⎤
15 Third ⎥ dorsal interosseous
16 Second ⎥
17 First ⎦
18 Extensor indicis
19 Extensor expansion

The anatomical snuffbox:
➤ When the thumb is extended fully the extensor tendons become taut at its base and bow-out to form a hollow depression (*the anatomical snuffbox*).
➤ It is formed laterally by the tendons of abductor pollicis longus and extensor pollicis brevis and medially by the tendon of extensor pollicis longus.

Adult bones of the left hand, palmar surface – *from the front*

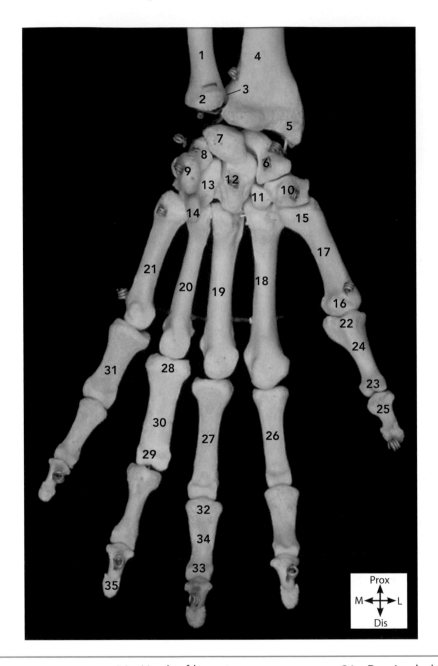

1 Shaft ⎤ of ulna	14 Hook of hamate	26 Proximal phalanx of index finger
2 Head ⎦	15 Base ⎤ of first (I)	27 Proximal phalanx of middle finger
3 Ulna notch	16 Head ⎟ metacarpal	
4 Shaft ⎫ of radius	17 Shaft ⎦ bone	28 Base ⎤ of proximal
5 Styloid process ⎭	18 Second (II) ⎤	29 Head ⎟ phalanx of
6 Scaphoid ⎤ proximal	19 Third (III) ⎟ metacarpal	30 Shaft ⎦ ring finger
7 Triquetral ⎟ row of	20 Fourth (IV) ⎟ bone	31 Proximal phalanx of little finger
8 Lunate ⎟ carpal bones	21 Fifth (V) ⎦	
9 Pisiform ⎦	22 Base ⎤ of proximal	32 Base ⎤ of middle
10 Trapezium ⎤ distal row	23 Head ⎟ phalanx	33 Head ⎟ phalanx of
11 Trapezoid ⎟ of carpal	24 Shaft ⎦ of thumb	34 Shaft ⎦ middle finger
12 Capitate ⎟ bones	25 Distal phalanx of thumb	35 Distal phalanx of ring finger
13 Hamate ⎦		

Adult bones of the left hand, dorsal surface – *from behind*

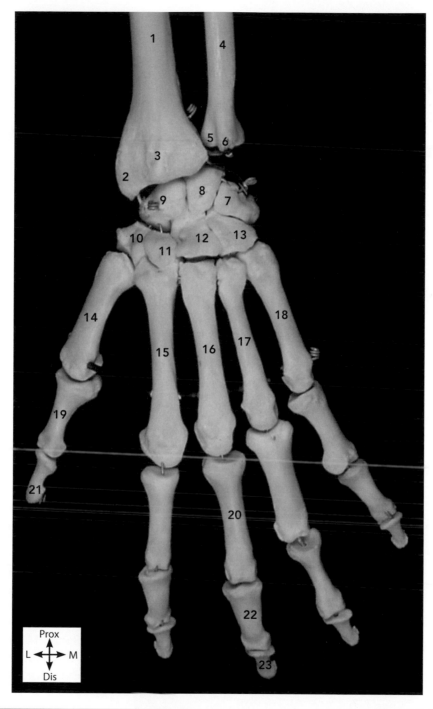

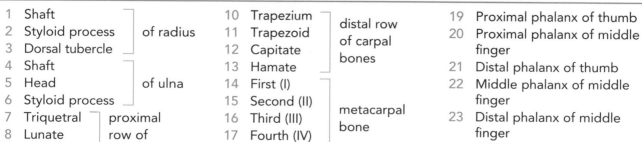

1	Shaft		10	Trapezium	19	Proximal phalanx of thumb
2	Styloid process	of radius	11	Trapezoid	distal row	20	Proximal phalanx of middle
3	Dorsal tubercle		12	Capitate	of carpal		finger
4	Shaft		13	Hamate	bones	21	Distal phalanx of thumb
5	Head	of ulna	14	First (I)		22	Middle phalanx of middle
6	Styloid process		15	Second (II)			finger
7	Triquetral	proximal	16	Third (III)	metacarpal	23	Distal phalanx of middle
8	Lunate	row of	17	Fourth (IV)	bone		finger
9	Scaphoid	carpal bones	18	Fifth (V)			

Coronal section through the left wrist joint and hand – *from behind*

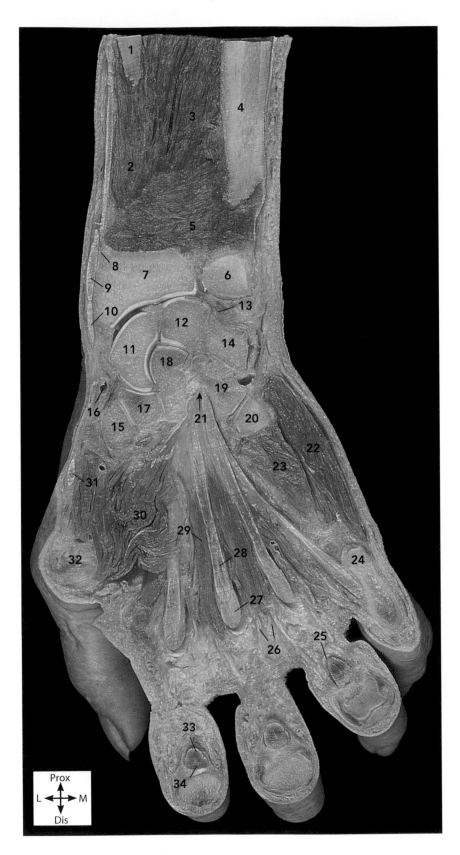

1 Shaft of radius
2 Flexor pollicis longus
3 Flexor digitorum profundus
4 Shaft of ulna
5 Pronator quadrates
6 Head of ulna
7 Distal end ⎤
8 Styloid process ⎦ of radius
9 Abductor pollicis longus
10 Extensor pollicis brevis
11 Scaphoid
12 Lunate
13 Articular disc (triangular fibrocartilaginous complex, TFCC)
14 Triquetral
15 Trapezium
16 Radial artery
17 Trapezoid
18 Capitate
19 Hamate
20 Base of fifth (V) metacarpal bone
21 Distal opening of carpal tunnel
22 Abductor digiti minimi
23 Flexor digitorum minimi
24 Base of proximal phalanx of little finger
25 Digital fibrous sheath of ring finger
26 Common digital artery and nerve
27 Tendon of flexor digitorum superficialis
28 Tendon of flexor digitorum profundus
29 Second lumbrical
30 Abductor pollicis
31 Extensor pollicis longus
32 Head of first (I) metacarpal bone
33 Tendon of flexor digitorum profundus ⎤ of index
34 Tendon of flexor digitorum superficialis ⎦ finger

Sagittal section through the joints of the left wrist and middle finger –
from the left

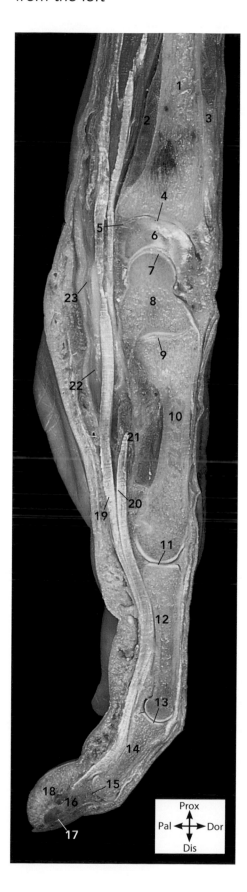

1 Shaft of radius
2 Pronator quadratus
3 Extensor digitorum
4 Radiocarpal joint (wrist joint)
5 Capsule of wrist joint
6 Lunate
7 Intercarpal joint
8 Capitate
9 Carpometacarpal joint
10 Third (III) metacarpal bone
11 Metacarpophalangeal joint
12 Proximal phalanx of middle finger
13 Interphalangeal joint
14 Middle phalanx of middle finger
15 Interphalangeal joint
16 Distal phalanx of middle finger
17 Nail bed
18 Pulp space of distal phalanx of middle finger
19 Tendon of flexor digitorum superficialis
20 Tendon of flexor digitorum profundus
21 Adductor pollicis
22 Palmar aponeurosis
23 Flexor retinaculum

The wrist joint:
➤ Is formed by three of the first row of carpal bones, the scaphoid, lunate and triquetral, which articulate with both the radius and articular (triangular) disc, hence its true name radiocarpal joint.
➤ Although the articular (triangular) disc joins the radius to the ulna, it also intervenes and separates the wrist joint from the distal radioulnar joint, thus the ulna does not form part of the wrist joint.

Superficial structures of the left forearm and palm of hand – *from the front*

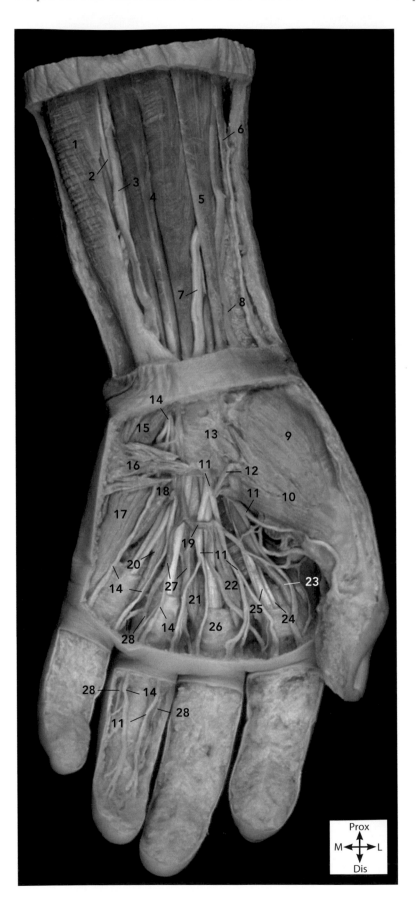

1 Flexor carpi ulnaris
2 Ulnar nerve
3 Ulnar artery
4 Flexor digitorum superficialis
5 Flexor carpi radialis
6 Brachioradialis
7 Median nerve
8 Radial artery
9 Abductor pollicis brevis
10 Flexor pollicis brevis
11 Digital branches ⎤
12 Recurrent branch ⎦ of median nerve
13 Flexor retinaculum
14 Digital branches of ulnar nerve
15 Abductor digiti minimi
16 Palmaris brevis
17 Flexor digiti minimi brevis
18 Opponens digiti minimi
19 Superficial palmar arch
20 Fourth ⎤
21 Third ⎥
22 Second ⎥ lumbrical
23 First ⎦
24 Tendon of flexor digitorum profundus
25 Tendon of flexor digitorum superficialis
26 Fibrous sheath of middle finger
27 Common palamar digital artery
28 Proper palmar digital artery

The flexor retinaculum:
➤ Is composed of tough fibrous tissue approximately 2 cm × 2.5 cm in area.
➤ It stretches between the scaphoid and trapezium on the radial side, and the hamate and pisiform bones on the ulnar side.
➤ It forms a roof over the carpal tunnel through which pass the long flexor tendons and the median nerve.
➤ The ulnar nerve and artery lie superficial to the flexor retinaculum.

Deep structures of the left distal forearm and palm of hand – *from the front*

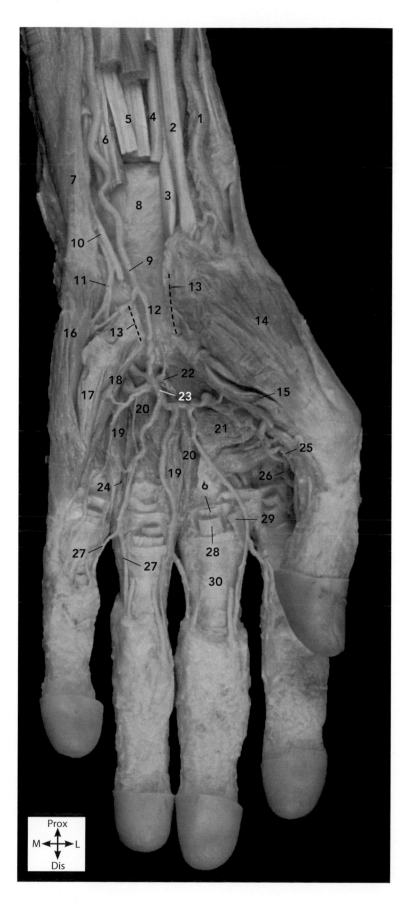

1 Radial artery
2 Flexor carpi radialis
3 Flexor pollicis longus
4 Median nerve
5 Flexor digitorum superficialis
6 Flexor digitorum profundus
7 Flexor carpi ulnaris
8 Fascia overlying pronator quadrates
9 Ulnar artery (superficial to removed flexor retinaculum)
10 Ulnar nerve
11 Superficial branch of ulnar nerve
12 Carpal tunnel (floor)
13 Cut edge of flexor retinaculum
14 Abductor pollicis brevis
15 Flexor pollicis brevis
16 Abductor digiti minimi
17 Flexor digiti minimi brevis
18 Opponens digiti minimi
19 Palmar interosseous
20 Dorsal interossei
21 Adductor pollicis
22 Deep palmar arch
23 Superficial palmar arch
24 Common palmar digital artery
25 Princeps pollicis artery
26 Radialis indicis artery
27 Proper palmar digital artery
28 Tendon of flexor digitorum superficialis
29 Second lumbrical
30 Fibrous flexor sheath

Deep structures of the left forearm and palm of hand – *from the front*

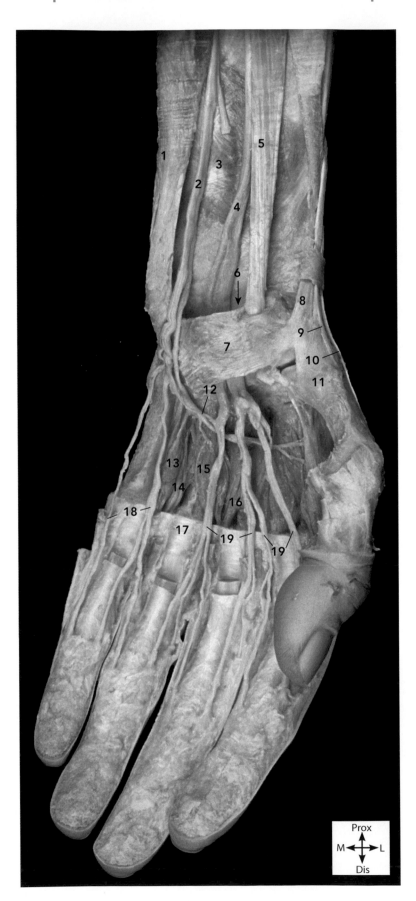

1   Flexor carpi ulnaris
2   Ulnar nerve
3   Pronator quadrates
4   Median nerve
5   Flexor carpi radialis
6   Carpal tunnel
7   Flexor retinaculum
8   Abductor pollicis longus
9   Extensor pollicis brevis
10 Extensor pollicis longus
11 Base of first (I) metacarpal bone
12 Deep branch of ulnar nerve
13 Third palmar ⎤
14 Fourth dorsal ⎥
15 Second palmar ⎥ interossei
16 Third dorsal ⎦
17 Deep transverse metacarpal ligament
18 Digital branches of ulnar nerve
19 Digital branches of median nerve

The ulnar nerve supplies:
➤ The lumbricals and interossei, muscles that provide delicate finger movements.
➤ The skin of the little finger and ulnar edge of the hand.

The median nerve supplies:
➤ The small muscles of the thumb, which are essential for the action of gripping.

Deep structures of the left distal forearm and palm of hand – *from the front*

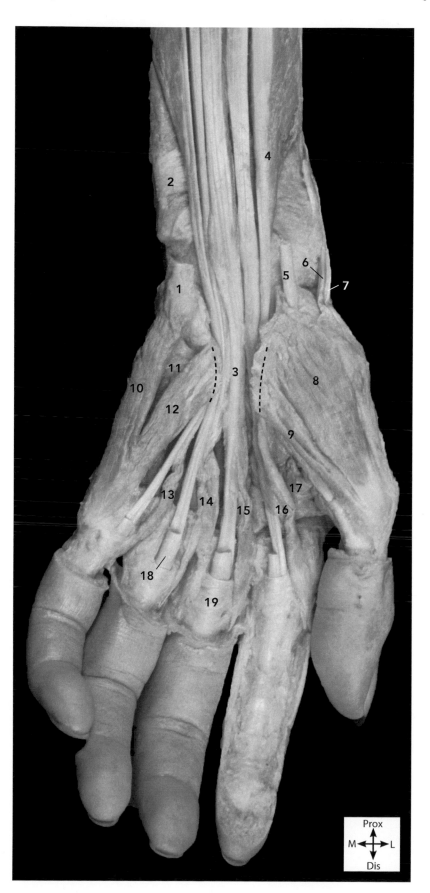

1 Tendon of flexor carpi ulnaris
2 Pronator quadrates
3 Tendons of flexor digitorum profundus within the carpal tunnel
4 Flexor pollicis longus
5 Tendon of flexor carpi radialis
6 Abductor pollicis longus
7 Extensor pollicis brevis
8 Abductor pollicis brevis
9 Flexor pollicis brevis
10 Abductor digiti minimi
11 Flexor digiti minimi brevis
12 Opponens digiti minimi
13 Fourth ⎤
14 Third ⎥ lumbrical
15 Second ⎥
16 First ⎦
17 Adductor pollicis
18 Tendon of flexor digitorum superficialis
19 Fibrous flexor sheath

Fibrous flexor sheaths:
➤ Form with the phalanges of each finger.
➤ Prevent the flexor tendons from bowing forwards when the fingers are flexed.

Synovial sheaths:
➤ Surround the tendons within the carpal tunnel and also within the fibrous sheaths of the fingers.
➤ Allow tendon movement without friction.

PART IV

Thorax

Adult right first (I) atypical rib – *A from above; B from below*

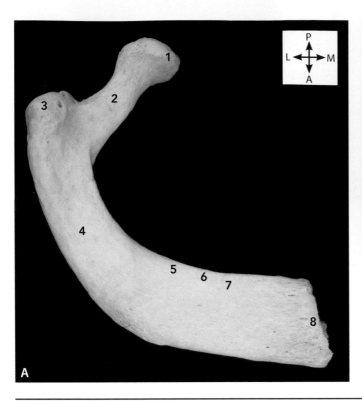

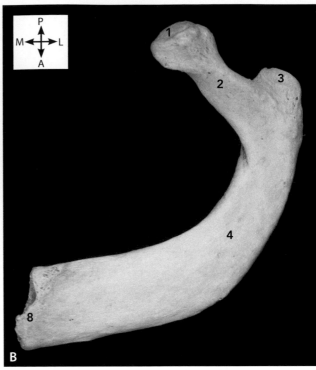

1	Head	4	Shaft	7	Groove for subclavian vein
2	Neck	5	Groove for subclavian artery	8	Anterior end
3	Tubercle	6	Scalene tubercle		

The first (I) rib:
➤ Is an atypical rib.
➤ Is the most curved, flattest and shortest of all the ribs.
➤ Articulates with only one vertebra, at its own level, the first (TI) thoracic vertebra.

Other atypical ribs are:
➤ The second (II), tenth (X), eleventh (XI) and twelfth (XII).

Adult right typical rib – *A from above; B from below*

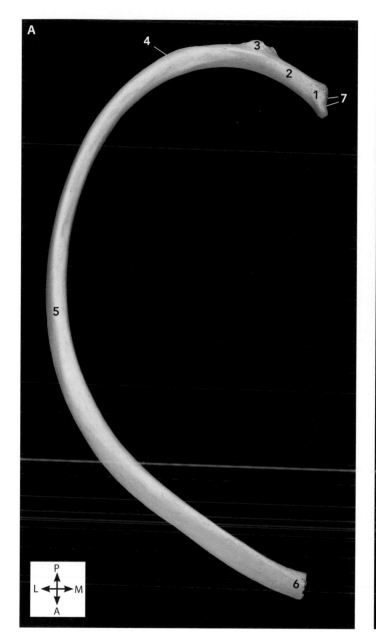

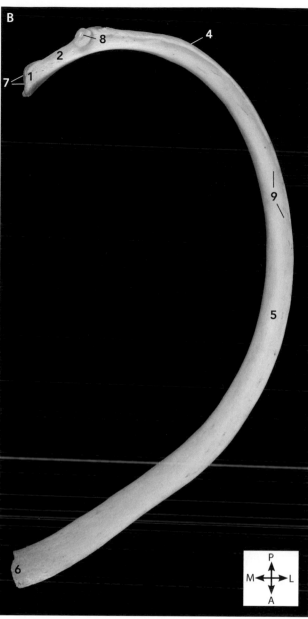

1	Head	4	Angle	7	Articular facet of head
2	Neck	5	Shaft	8	Articular facet of tubercle
3	Tubercle	6	Anterior end	9	Costal groove

The seven typical ribs are the third to ninth (III–IX):

➤ Have a head with two facets and a tubercle that has both articular and non-articular parts; the facets and tubercle are situated each end of the ribs neck and articulate with the body of two separate vertebra, one at the rib's own level and the one above.

➤ For example, the fifth (V) rib articulates with the body of the fifth (TV) thoracic vertebra and also the body of the one above, the fourth (TIV) thoracic vertebra.

Adult skeleton of the thorax – *from the front*

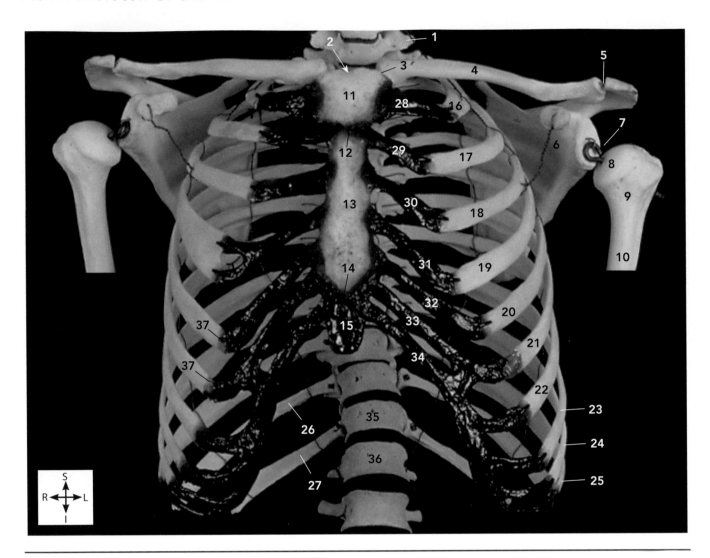

1	Seventh (CVII) cervical vertebra – vertebra prominens	14	Xiphisternal joint	28 First
2	Suprasternal notch	15	Xiphoid process of sternum	29 Second
3	Sternoclavicular joint	16	First (I)	30 Third
4	Body of clavicle	17	Second (II)	31 Fourth costal cartilage
5	Acromioclavicular joint	18	Third (III)	32 Fifth
6	Scapula	19	Fourth (IV)	33 Sixth
7	Shoulder joint	20	Fifth (V)	34 Seventh
8	Head	21	Sixth (VI)	35 Twelfth (TXII) thoracic vertebra
9	Surgical neck of humerus	22	Seventh (VII) rib	36 First (LI) lumbar vertebra
10	Shaft	23	Eighth (VIII)	37 Costochondral junction
11	Manubrium of sternum	24	Ninth (IX)	
12	Manubriosternal joint	25	Tenth (X)	
13	Body of sternum	26	Eleventh (XI)	
		27	Twelfth (XII)	

The ribs are defined as:
➤ The seven true ribs, the first to seventh (I–VII): are joined to the sternum by their costal cartilages.
➤ The five false ribs, the eighth to twelfth (VIII–XII): are joined by their cartilages to the cartilage above.
➤ The two floating ribs, eleventh and twelfth (XI, XII): are short and are not joined to others.

Muscles of the external thoracic wall – *from the front*

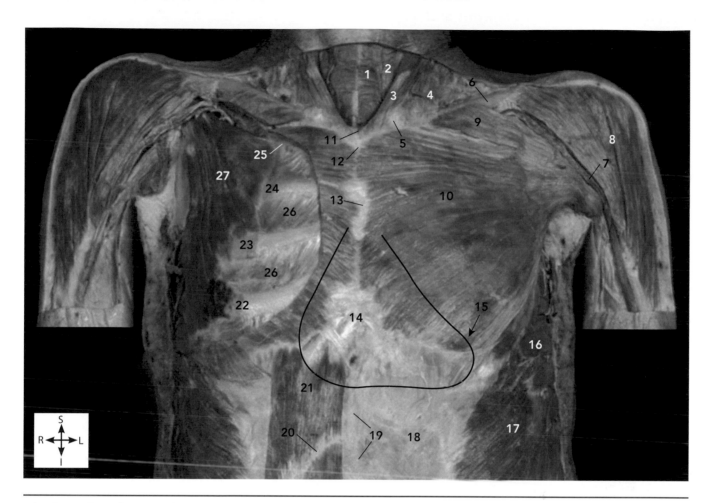

1	Sternohyoid	15	Approximate position of heart (outlined)
2	Sternothyroid	16	Serratus anterior
3	Sternal ⎤ head of sternocleidomastoid	17	External oblique
4	Clavicular ⎦	18	Rectus sheath
5	Capsule of sternoclavicular joint	19	Linea alba
6	Body of clavicle	20	Tendinous intersection of rectus abdominis
7	Cephalic vein in deltopectoral groove	21	Rectus abdominis
8	Deltoid	22	Fourth (IV) ⎤
9	Clavicular ⎤ part of pectoralis major	23	Third (III) ⎥ rib
10	Sternocostal ⎦	24	Second (II) ⎥
11	Suprasternal notch	25	First (I) ⎦
12	Manubrium ⎤	26	External intercostals
13	Body ⎥ of sternum	27	Pectoralis minor
14	Xiphoid process ⎦		

Superficial structures of the female breast and external thoracic wall – *from the front and left*

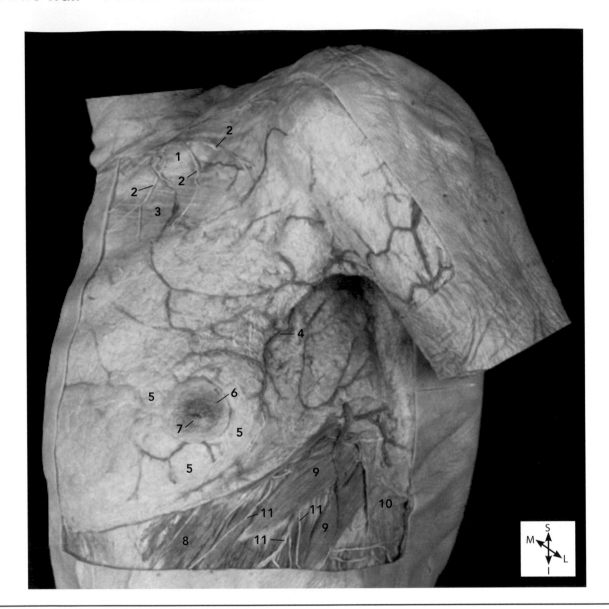

1	Fascia overlying body of clavicle	4	Branches of lateral thoracic artery	8	External oblique
2	Supraclavicular nerves	5	Fat	9	Serratus anterior
3	Fascia overlying pectoralis major	6	Areola } of breast	10	Latissimus dorsi
		7	Nipple	11	Cutaneous branches of intercostal nerves

The female breast:
➤ Is situated in the subcutaneous tissue of the anterior thoracic wall.
➤ Mainly comprises variable amounts of fat, which provides the bulk of the breasts volume; within the fat is a framework of fibrous tissue and ducts.
➤ Main part of the breast overlays pectoralis major.
➤ Base of the breast, which is constant in position, extends from near the midline to the midaxillary line, and from the second (II) to the sixth (VI) rib.
➤ Main blood supply to the breast is from the internal thoracic artery and adjacent intercostal vessels.
➤ Lactiferous ducts, about 15 in number, communicate with and open at the nipple.

Sagittal section through the left female breast – *from the left*

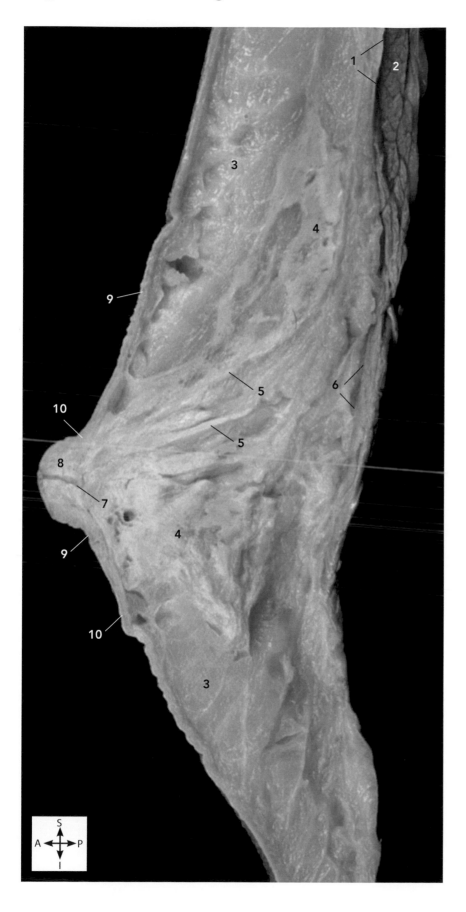

1 Fascia overlying pectoralis major
2 Pectoralis major
3 Fat of breast
4 Condensed glandular tissue
5 Fibrous septum (suspensory ligaments)
6 Retromammary space
7 Lactiferous duct
8 Nipple ⎤ of breast
9 Areola ⎦
10 Skin and subcutaneous tissue of breast

Lymphatic drainage of the breast:
➤ Is mostly to the axillary group of lymph nodes (which may be palpable).
➤ Can also pass through drainage channels that pass through the chest wall to the parasternal group of lymph nodes (which are not palpable), situated within the thorax beside the internal thoracic vessels.

Thorax with ribcage and thoracic viscera *in situ* – *from the front*

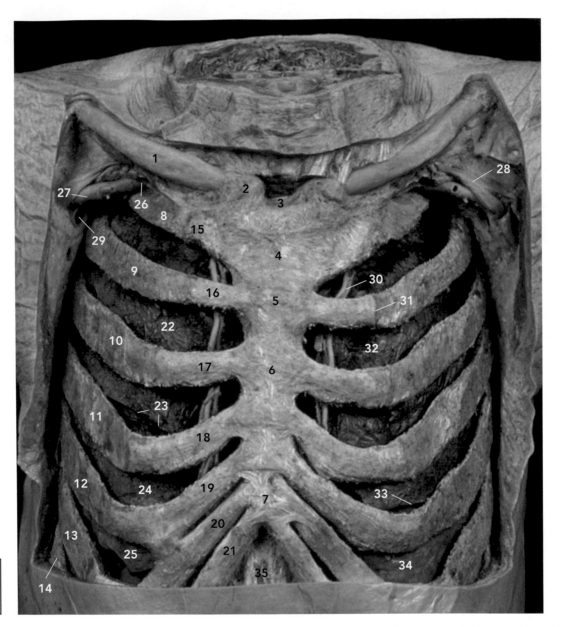

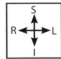

1	Body of clavicle	15	First	29	Axillary vein
2	Capsule of sternoclavicular joint	16	Second	30	Internal thoracic artery and vein
3	Suprasternal notch	17	Third	costal cartilage	
4	Manubrium of sternum	18	Fourth		31 Costochondral junction
5	Manubriosternal joint	19	Fifth		32 Superior lobe ⎤ of left lung
6	Body ⎤ of sternum	20	Sixth		33 Oblique fissure ⎦
7	Xiphoid process ⎦	21	Seventh		34 Superior surface of left dome of diaphragm
8	First (I)	22	Superior lobe		35 Central tendon of diaphragm
9	Second (II)	23	Transverse fissure	of right lung	
10	Third (III)	24	Middle lobe		
11	Fourth (IV) rib	25	Inferior lobe		
12	Fifth (IV)	26	Subclavian artery		
13	Sixth (VI)	27	Axillary artery		
14	Seventh (VII)	28	Brachial plexus		

Thorax with ribcage removed and thoracic viscera *in situ* – *from the front*

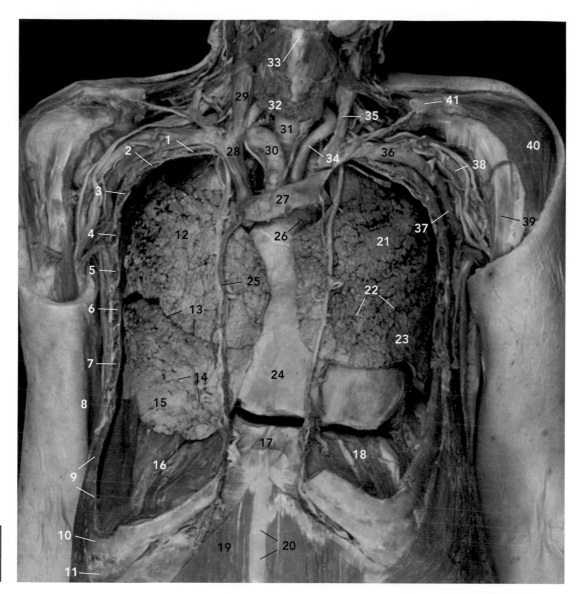

1	First (I)	16	Superior surface of right dome of diaphragm	29	Right internal jugular vein
2	Second (II)			30	Brachiocephalic trunk
3	Third (III)	17	Central tendon of diaphragm	31	Trachea
4	Fourth (IV)	18	Superior surface of left dome of diaphragm	32	Right lobe of thyroid gland
5	Fifth (V) rib			33	Laryngeal prominence of thyroid cartilage
6	Sixth (VI)	19	Rectus abdominis		
7	Seventh (VII)	20	Linea alba	34	Left common carotid artery
8	Eight (VIII)	21	Superior lobe	35	Left internal jugular vein
9	Ninth (IX)	22	Oblique fissure of left lung	36	Subclavian vein
10	Ninth costal	23	Inferior lobe	37	Axillary vein
11	Tenth cartilage	24	Pericardium (pericardial sac)	38	Axillary artery
12	Superior lobe	25	Internal thoracic artery and vein	39	Long head of biceps
13	Transverse fissure of right			40	Deltoid
14	Oblique fissure lung	26	Arch of aorta	41	Body of clavicle
15	Inferior lobe	27	Left brachiocephalic		
		28	Right vein		

Right lung, lateral aspect – *from the right*

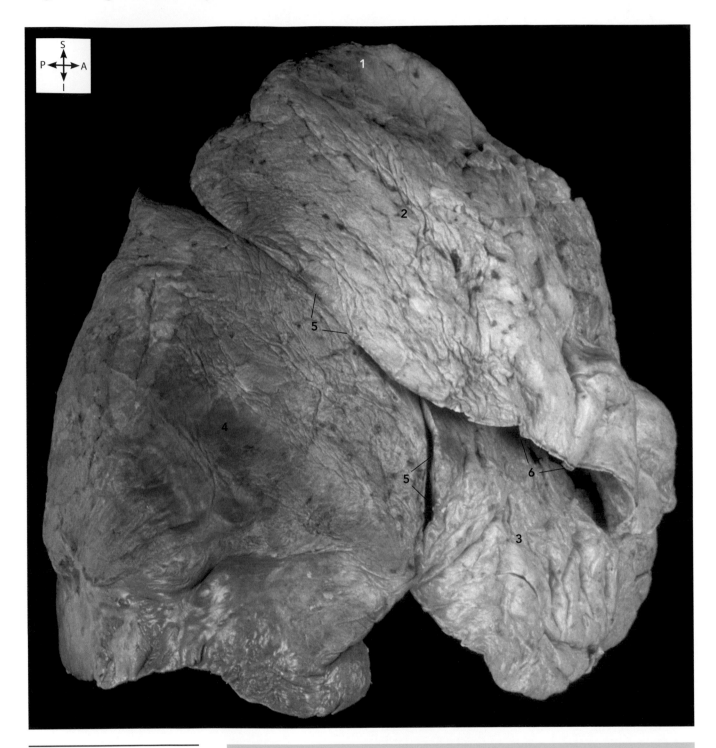

1	Apex
2	Superior lobe
3	Middle lobe
4	Inferior lobe
5	Oblique fissure
6	Transverse fissure

Bronchopulmonary segments of the three lobes of the right lung are:

➤ **Superior lobe:**
Apical segment (SI)
Posterior segment (SII)
Anterior segment (SIII)

➤ **Middle lobe:**
Lateral segment (SIV)
Medial segment (SV)

➤ **Inferior lobe:**
Apical (superior) (SVI)
Medial basal (SVII)
Anterior basal (SVIII)
Lateral basal (SIX)
Posterior basal (SX)

Left lung, lateral aspect – *from the right*

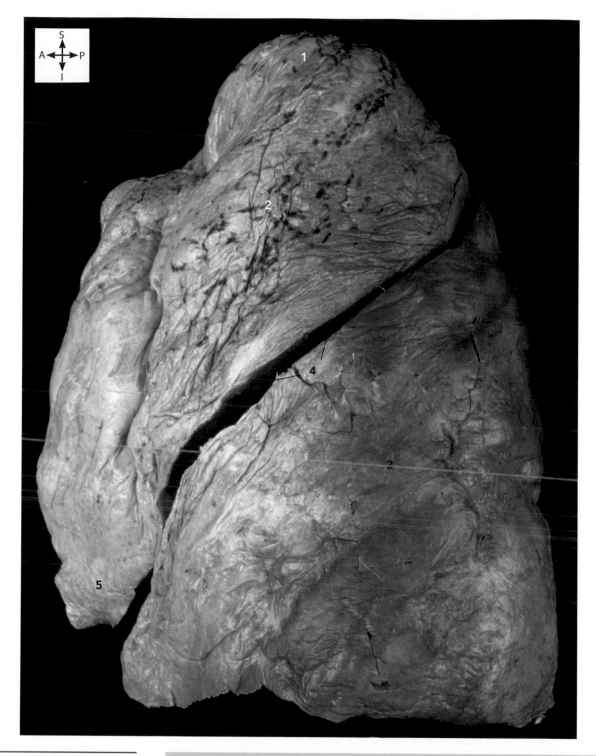

1	Apex
2	Superior lobe
3	Inferior lobe
4	Oblique fissure
5	Lingula

Bronchopulmonary segments of the two lobes of the left lung are:

➤ **Superior lobe:**

Apicoposterior segment
  (SI + SII)

Anterior segment (SIII)

Superior lingular segment (SIV)

Inferior lingular segment (SV)

➤ **Inferior lobe:**

Superior segment (SVI)

Medial basal (SVII)

Anterior basal (SVIII)

Lateral basal (SIX)

Posterior basal (SX)

Right lung, medial aspect – *from the left*

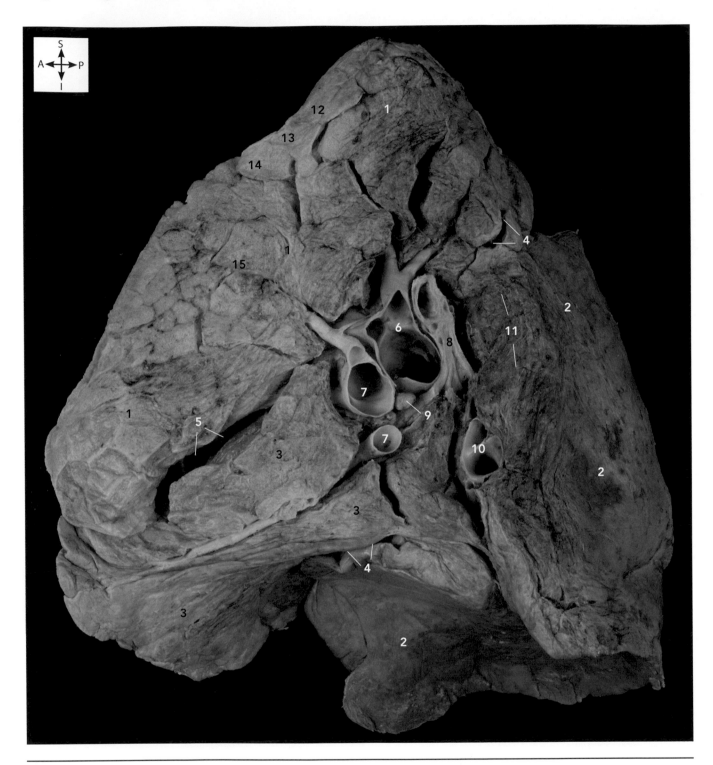

1	Superior		6	Right pulmonary artery (divided)
2	Inferior	lobe	7	Right superior pulmonary veins
3	Middle		8	Right main bronchus (divided)
4	Oblique	fissure	9	Hilar lymph nodes
5	Transverse		10	Right inferior pulmonary veins

11 Groove for azygos vein
12 Groove for subclavian artery
13 Groove for subclavian vein
14 Groove for first (I) rib
15 Groove for superior vena cava

Right lung root and mediastinum – *from the right*

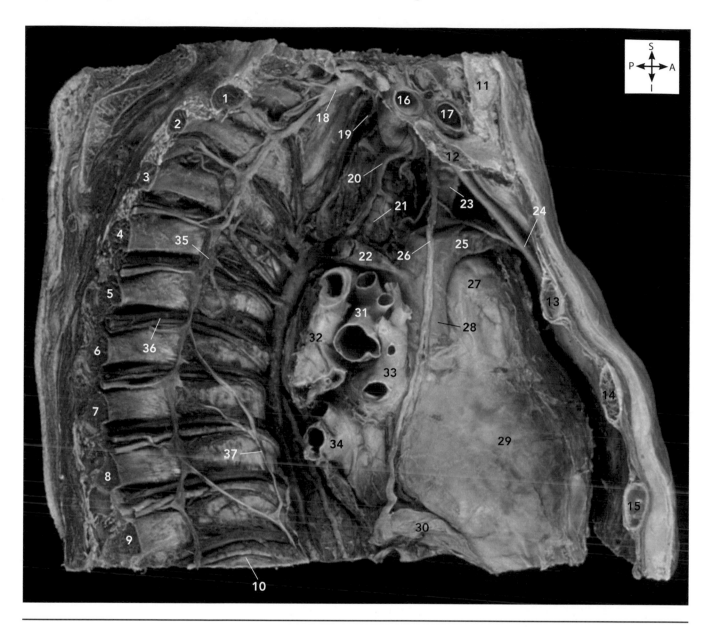

1	First (I)	16	Right subclavian artery
2	Second (II)	17	Right subclavian vein
3	Third (III)	18	Cervicothoracic (stellate) ganglion
4	Fourth (IV)	19	Oesophagus
5	Fifth (V) rib	20	Vagus nerve
6	Sixth (VI)	21	Trachea
7	Seventh (VII)	22	Azygos vein
8	Eighth (VIII)	23	Right brachiocephalic vein
9	Ninth (IX)	24	Internal thoracic artery and vein
10	Tenth (X)	25	Left brachiocephalic vein
11	Body of clavicle	26	Phrenic nerve
12	First	27	Pericardium covering ascending aorta
13	Second costal cartilage	28	Superior vena cava
14	Third		
15	Fourth		

29 Pericardium (pericardial sac) over right atrium
30 Superior surface (floor) of right dome of diaphragm
31 Right pulmonary artery (divided)
32 Right main bronchus (divided)
33 Right superior pulmonary vein (divided)
34 Right inferior pulmonary vein (divided)
35 Sympathetic trunk and ganglion
36 Posterior intercostal artery, vein and nerve
37 Greater splanchnic nerve

Left lung root and mediastinum – *from the left*

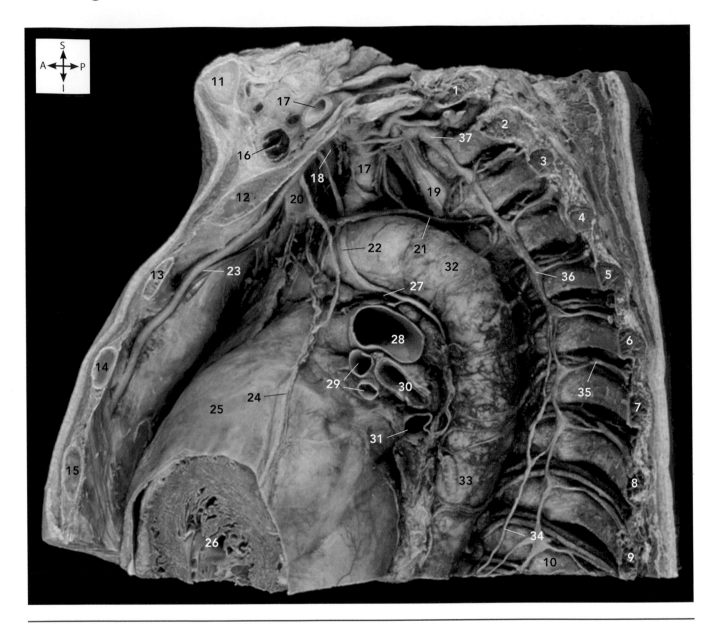

1	First (I) ⎤	16 Left subclavian vein
2	Second (II)	17 Left subclavian artery
3	Third (III)	18 Left common carotid artery
4	Fourth (IV)	19 Oesophagus
5	Fifth (V) rib	20 Left brachiocephalic vein
6	Sixth (VI)	21 Superior intercostal vein
7	Seventh (VII)	22 Vagus nerve
8	Eighth (VIII)	23 Internal thoracic artery and vein
9	Ninth (IX)	24 Phrenic nerve
10	Tenth (X) ⎦	25 Pericardium (pericardial sac)
11	Body of clavicle	26 Left ventricle of heart
12	First ⎤	27 Recurrent laryngeal nerve
13	Second	costal cartilage	28 Left pulmonary artery
14	Third		29 Left superior pulmonary vein (divided)
15	Fourth ⎦	

30 Left main bronchus
31 Left inferior pulmonary vein
32 Arch of aorta
33 Descending thoracic aorta
34 Greater splanchnic nerve
35 Posterior intercostal artery, vein and nerve
36 Sympathetic trunk and ganglion
37 Cervicothoracic (stellate) ganglion

Left lung, medial aspect – *from the right*

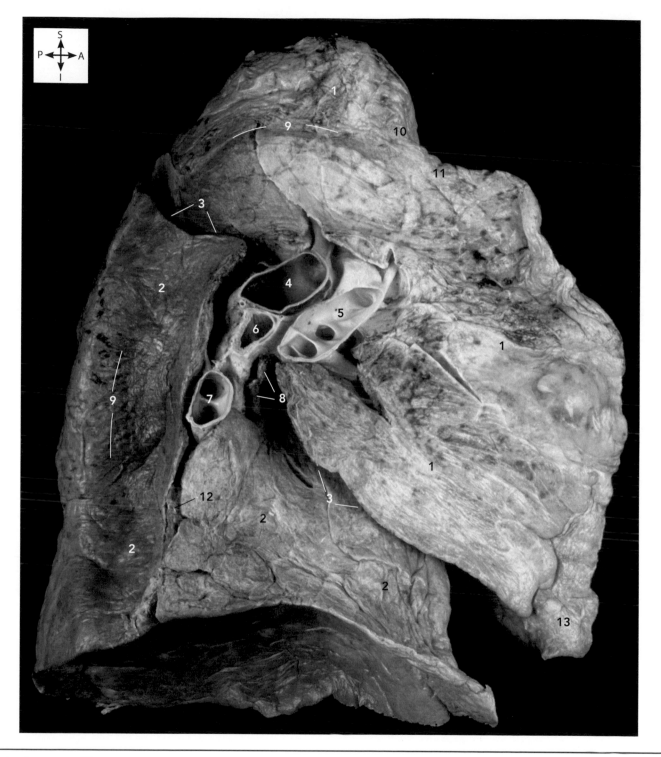

1	Superior ⎤ lobe	8	Hilar lymph nodes
2	Inferior ⎦	9	Groove for aorta
3	Oblique fissure	10	Groove for left subclavian artery
4	Left pulmonary artery	11	Groove for first (I) rib
5	Left superior pulmonary veins (divided)	12	Pulmonary ligament
6	Left main bronchus	13	Lingula
7	Left inferior pulmonary veins (divided)		

Heart – *from the front*

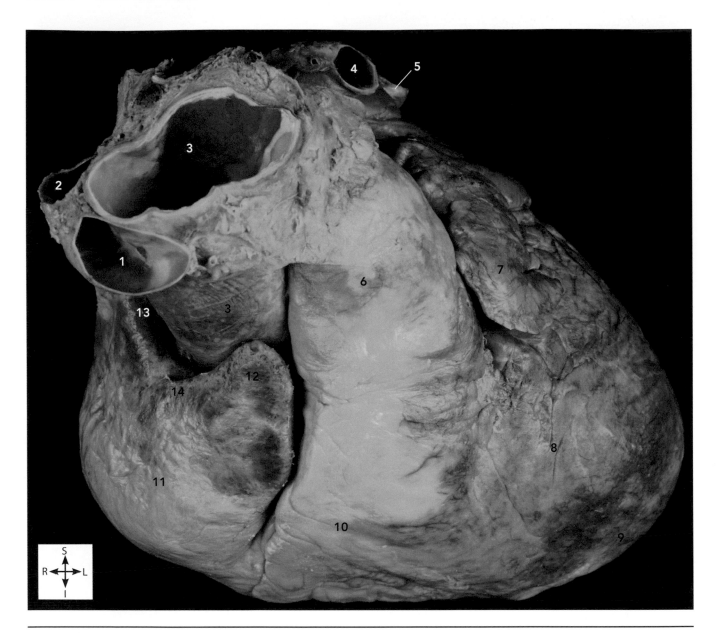

1	Left ⎤ brachiocephalic vein	8	Left ventricle
2	Right ⎦	9	Apex
3	Ascending aorta	10	Right ventricle
4	Left superior ⎤ pulmonary vein	11	Right atrium
5	Left inferior ⎦	12	Auricle of right atrium
6	Pulmonary trunk	13	Superior vena cava
7	Auricle of left atrium	14	Position of sinu–atrial (SA) node in atrial wall

Heart, superficial structures – *from the front*

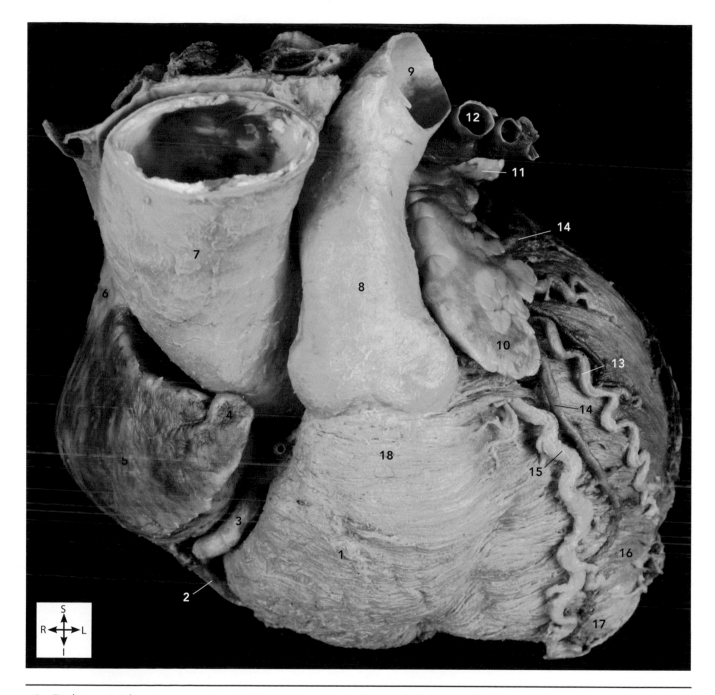

1 Right ventricle	11 Left inferior ⎤ pulmonary vein
2 Small cardiac vein	12 Left superior ⎦
3 Right coronary artery in atrioventricular groove	13 Marginal branch of left coronary artery
4 Auricle of right atrium	14 Great cardiac vein
5 Right atrium	15 Anterior interventricular branch of left coronary artery in interventricular groove
6 Superior vena cava	
7 Ascending aorta	16 Left ventricle
8 Pulmonary trunk	17 Apex
9 Left pulmonary artery	18 Infundibulum of right ventricle
10 Auricle of left atrium	

Heart – *from behind*

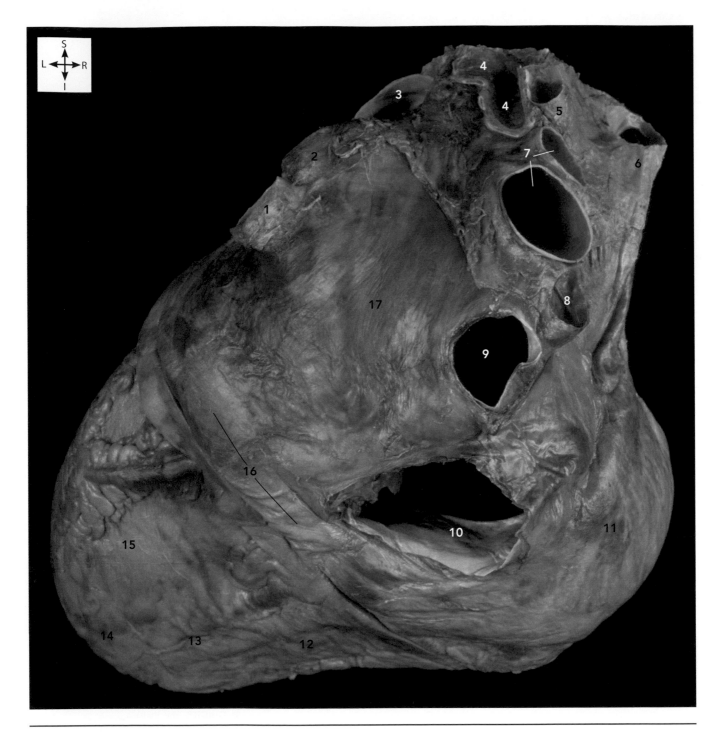

1 Left inferior ⎤ pulmonary	8 Right superior ⎤ pulmonary	14 Apex
2 Left superior ⎦ vein	9 Right inferior ⎦ vein	15 Left ventricular wall
3 Left pulmonary artery	10 Inferior vena cava	16 Coronary sinus in
4 Left and right main bronchus	11 Right atrium	atrioventricular groove
5 Azygos vein	12 Right ventricular wall	17 Left atrium
6 Superior vena cava	13 Position of interventricular	
7 Right pulmonary artery (divided)	groove	

Heart, superficial structures – *from behind*

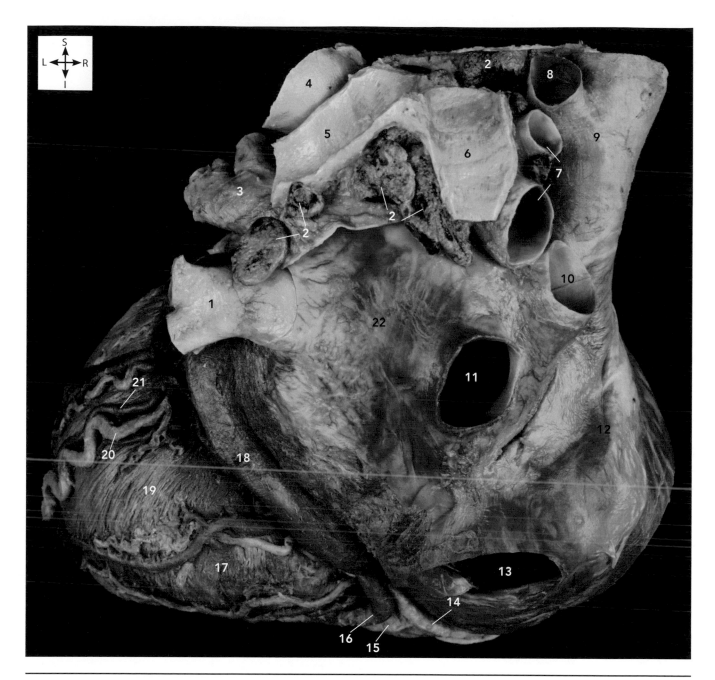

1	Left inferior pulmonary vein	
2	Trachiobronchial lymph nodes	
3	Left superior pulmonary vein	
4	Left pulmonary artery	
5	Left ⎤ main bronchus	
6	Right ⎦	
7	Right pulmonary artery (divided)	
8	Azygos vein	
9	Superior vena cava	
10	Right superior ⎤ pulmonary	
11	Right inferior ⎦ vein	
12	Right atrium	
13	Inferior vena cava	
14	Right coronary artery in atrioventricular groove	
15	Posterior interventricular branch of right coronary artery	
16	Middle cardiac vein in posterior interventricular groove	
17	Right ventricle	
18	Coronary sinus in atrioventricular (coronary) groove	
19	Left ventricle	
20	Circumflex branch of the left coronary artery	
21	Left posterior ventricular vein	
22	Left atrium	

Heart, bisected by coronal section, anterior half – *from behind*

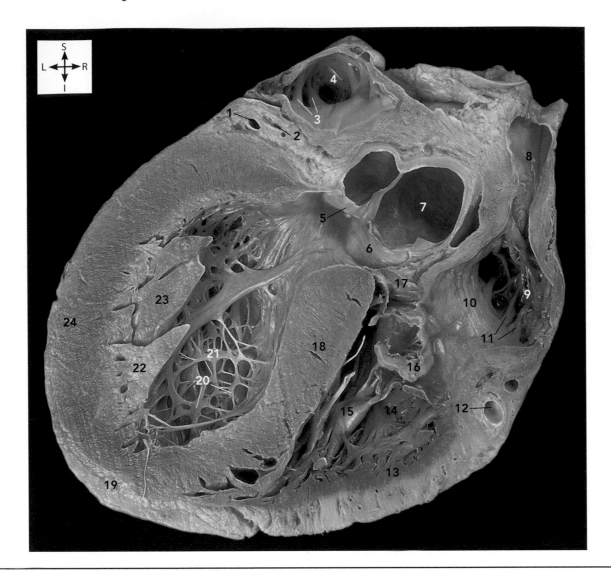

1	Great cardiac vein	13	Right ventricular wall
2	Branches of left coronary artery	14	Right ventricle
3	Musculi pectinati in left auricle	15	Anterior papillary muscle in right ventricle
4	Left auricle	16	Anterior cusp of tricuspid valve
5	Left cusp ⎤ of aortic valve	17	Membranous part of interventricular septum
6	Right cusp ⎦	18	Interventricular septum
7	Ascending aorta	19	Apex
8	Superior vena cava	20	Trabeculae carnae in left ventricle
9	Right auricle	21	Left ventricle
10	Right atrium	22	Posterior papillary ⎤ muscle of left ventricle
11	Musculi pectinati in right auricle	23	Anterior papillary ⎦
12	Right coronary artery in atrioventricular groove	24	Left ventricular wall

Blood flow via the chambers of the heart:
➤ The **right atrium** receives venous blood from the superior vena cava and the main vein of the heart (the coronary sinus).
➤ It then flows through the tricuspid valve into the **right ventricle**.
➤ Then through the pulmonary valve and into the pulmonary trunk (right and left pulmonary arteries) taking **deoxygenated blood** to the lungs.

Heart, bisected by coronal section, posterior half – *from the front*

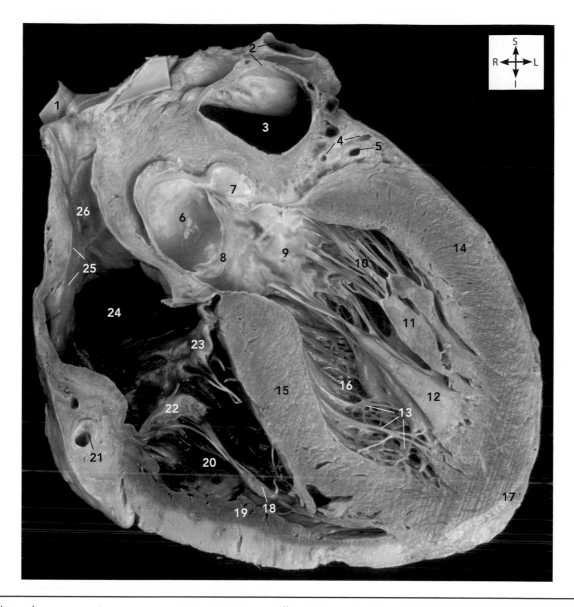

1 Right pulmonary veins	11 Anterior papillary ⎤ muscle of	20 Right ventricle
2 Left pulmonary veins entering left atrium	12 Posterior papillary ⎦ left ventricle	21 Right coronary artery in atrioventricular groove
3 Left atrium	13 Trabeculae carnae in left ventricle	22 Posterior cusp ⎤ of tricuspid
4 Left coronary artery branches	14 Left ventricular wall	23 Septal cusp ⎦ valve
5 Great cardiac vein	15 Interventricular septum	24 Right atrium
6 Ascending aorta	16 Left ventricle	25 Crista terminalis
7 Left cusp ⎤ of aortic	17 Apex	26 Superior vena cava
8 Posterior cusp ⎦ valve	18 Posterior papillary muscle of right ventricle	
9 Anterior cusp of mitral valve	19 Right ventricular wall	
10 Chordae tendinae		

Oxygenated blood from the lungs:
➤ Flows via the pulmonary veins into the **left atrium** and passes through the (bicuspid) mitral valve and into the **left ventricle**.
➤ Then through the aortic valve to enter the **aorta**, the body's largest blood vessel.

Heart, with right atrium exposed – *from the front and slightly right*

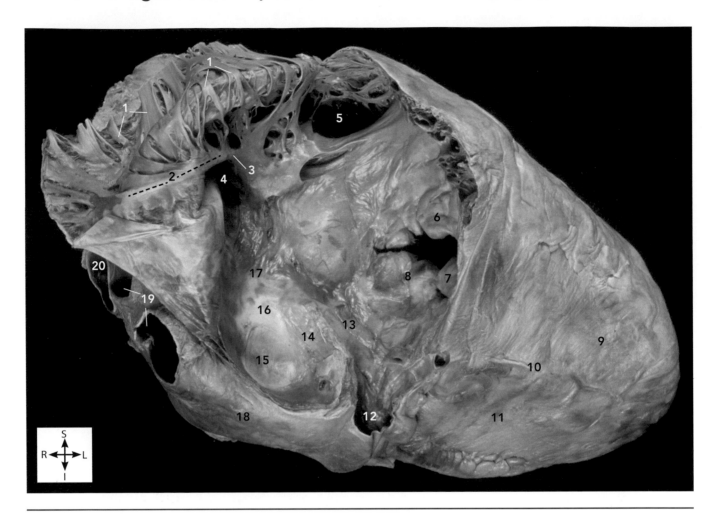

1	Musculi pectinati	9	Right ventricular wall	16	Position of intravenous tubercle of interatrial septum
2	Crista terminalis	10	Position of interventricular groove	17	Interatrial septum
3	Position of sinu-atrial (SA) node	11	Left ventricular wall	18	Left atrium
4	Superior vena cava	12	Coronary sinus	19	Right pulmonary veins
5	Right auricle	13	Position of atrioventricular (AV) node	20	Right pulmonary artery
6	Anterior cusp ⎤	14	Limbus fossa ovalis		
7	Posterior cusp ⎥ of tricuspid valve	15	Fossa ovalis		
8	Septal cusp ⎦				

The right and left atria:
➤ Are separated by the interatrial septum.

The right and left ventricles:
➤ Are separated by the interventricular septum.

Heart valves: pulmonary (*open*), aortic (*closed*) and mitral (*closed*), *in situ* –
from above

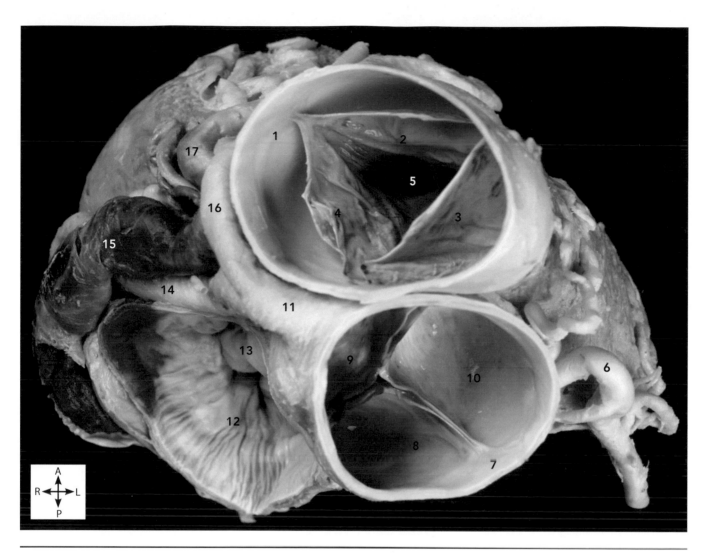

1 Pulmonary trunk
2 Left cusp ⎤ of open
3 Right cusp ⎥ pulmonary
4 Posterior cusp ⎦ valve
5 Right ventricle
6 Right coronary artery in atrioventricular groove
7 Ascending aorta

8 Posterior cusp ⎤ of closed
9 Left cusp ⎥ aortic valve
10 Right cusp ⎦
11 Posterior interventricular artery in interventricular groove
12 Posterior cusp ⎤ of closed
13 Anterior cusp ⎦ mitral valve

14 Circumflex branch of left coronary artery
15 Coronary sinus in atrioventricular (coronary) groove
16 Anterior interventricular branch of left coronary artery in interventricular groove
17 Great cardiac vein

The four main chambers of the heart and associated valves are:
➤ Pumping **deoxygenated blood** to the lungs:
  ➤ Right atrium – tricuspid valve.
  ➤ Right ventricle – pulmonary valve.
➤ Pumping (drawing) **oxygenated blood** from the lungs:
  ➤ Left atrium – mitral valve.
  ➤ Left ventricle – aortic valve.
➤ The tricuspid, pulmonary and aortic valves have **three cusps**.
➤ The mitral valve has **two cusps**.

Diaphragm, superior surface (thoracic floor) – *from above*

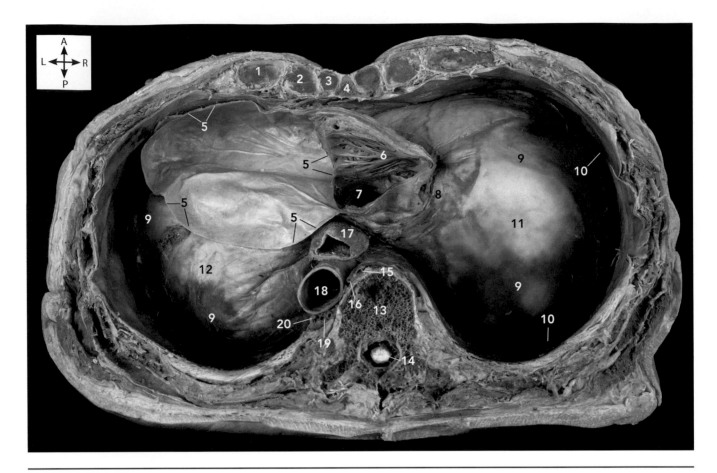

1	Fifth ⎤ costal cartilage	6	Musculi pectinati of right atrium	14	Spinal medulla (spinal cord) within vertebral canal
2	Sixth ⎦	7	Inferior vena cava	15	Azygos vein
3	Costal margin, united cartilages eminating from ribs seven (VII), eight (VII), nine (IX) and ten (X)	8	Central tendon of diaphragm	16	Thoracic duct
		9	Muscle of diaphragm	17	Oesophagus
		10	Diaphragmatic recess	18	Thoracic aorta
4	Xiphoid process of sternum	11	Right ⎤ superior surface of	19	Hemi-azygos vein
5	Pericardium, cut edge of pericardial sac	12	Left ⎦ dome of diaphragm	20	Greater splanchnic nerve
		13	Body of tenth (TX) thoracic vertebra		

The diaphragm:
➤ Forms a domed-shaped muscular and tendinous partition between the thorax and abdomen.
➤ Has a vertebral part with attachments to the first three lumbar vertebra; from the first (LI) and second (LII), which form the left crus and from the the first (LI), second (LII) and third (LIII) which form the right crus. Thickened fascia covering both the psoas major and quadrates lumborum muscles form a series of fibrous arches (the arcuate ligaments).
➤ Has a costal part with attachments to the inner surfaces of the first six (I-VI) ribs and the xiphoid process of the sternum, from which muscle fibres converge to form the (trefoil) structure of the central tendon which fuses with the pericardium.
➤ Has three main openings.

Diaphragm, inferior surface (abdominal roof) – *from below*

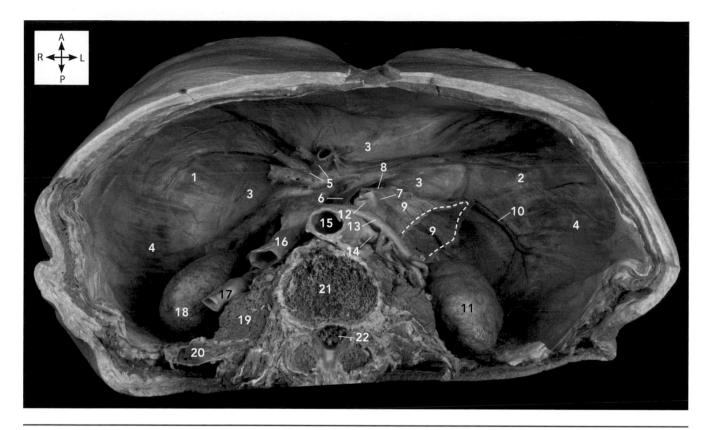

1	Right ⎤ inferior surface of	9	Fundus of stomach	17	Gonadal vein (enlarged)
2	Left ⎦ dome of diaphragm	10	Inferior phrenic vessels	18	Lower pole of right kidney
3	Central tendon of diaphragm	11	Lower pole of left kidney	19	Psoas major
4	Muscle of diaphragm	12	Coeliac trunk	20	Quadratus lumborum
5	Hepatic vessels	13	Left renal vein	21	Body of third (LIII) lumbar
6	Right ⎤ crus of diaphragm	14	Left renal artery		vertebra
7	Left ⎦	15	Abdominal aorta	22	Cauda equina within vertebral
8	Oesophagus	16	Inferior vena cava		canal

The diaphragms three main openings and nerve supply:

➤ **Aortic opening** – behind the crura at the level of the twelfth (TXII) thoracic vertebra, for passage of the aorta, thoracic duct and often the azygos vein.

➤ **Oesophageal opening** – in the muscle fibres of the right crus, just to the left of the midline at the level of the tenth (TX) thoracic vertebra, for passage of the oesophagus, branches of the left gastric vessels and vagal trunk.

➤ **Vena caval opening** – within the tendon at the level of the intervertebral disc between the eighth (TVIII) and ninth (TIX) thoracic vertebra, for passage of the inferior vena cava and right phrenic nerve.

➤ **The phrenic nerves** are the main motor supply to the diaphragm.

PART V

Abdomen and Pelvis

Adult skeleton of the abdominal region – *from the front*

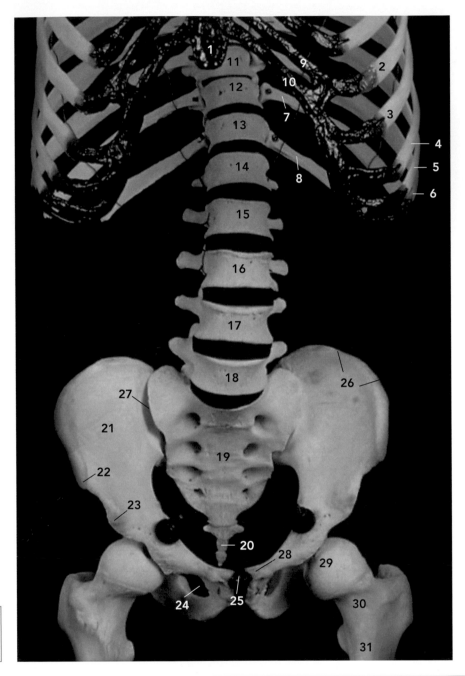

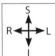

1	Xiphoid process	11	Tenth (TX)	22	Anterior superior ⎤ iliac
2	Sixth (VI) ⎤	12	Eleventh (TXI) thoracic vertebra	23	Anterior inferior ⎦ spine
3	Seventh (VII)	13	Twelfth (TXII)	24	Obturator foramen
4	Eighth (VIII)	14	First (LI) ⎤	25	Pubic symphysis
5	Ninth (IX) rib	15	Second (LII)	26	Iliac crest
6	Tenth (X)	16	Third (LIII) lumbar vertebra	27	Sacro-iliac joint
7	Eleventh (XI)	17	Fourth (LIV)	28	Pubic tubercle
8	Twelfth (XII) ⎦	18	Fifth (LV) ⎦	29	Head ⎤
9	Sixth ⎤ costal cartilage	19	Sacrum (sacral vertebrae I–V)	30	Neck ⎥ of femur
10	Seventh ⎦	20	Coccyx (coccygeal vertebrae I–IV)	31	Shaft ⎦
		21	Hip bone		

Abdomen, muscles of the anterior wall – *from the front*

The nine regions of the abdomen:

A Upper central – **epigastric region**
B Central   – **umbilical region**
C Lower central – **pubic region**

D Right – **hypochondrium** – left
E Right – **lateral (flank) region** – left
F Right – **inguinal (groin) region** – left

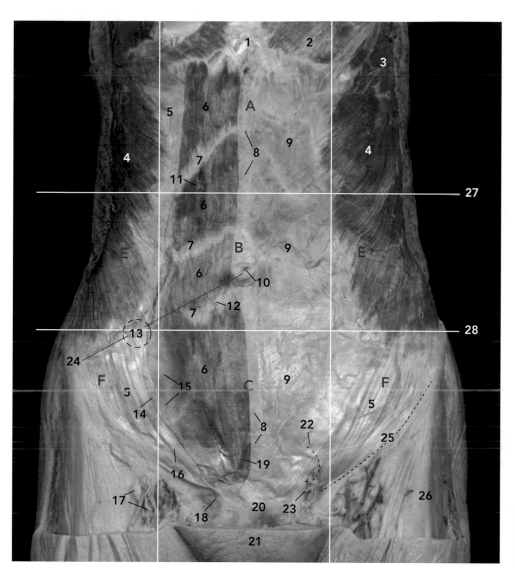

McBurney's point:
➤ Is an important site locatable on the surface of the anterior abdominal wall.
➤ It identifies the usual internal location of the base of the appendix.
➤ The point lies one-third of the way along a direct line from the right anterior superior iliac spine of the hip bone to the umbilicus.

1	Xiphoid process of sternum	
2	Sternocostal part of pectoralis major	
3	Serratus anterior	
4	External oblique	
5	External oblique aponeurosis	
6	Rectus abdominis	
7	Tendinous intersection of rectus abdominis	
8	Linea alba	
9	Rectus sheath	
10	Umbilicus	
11	Anterior cutaneous nerve (eighth intercostal)	
12	Anterior cutaneous nerve (tenth intercostal)	
13	McBurney's point (circled)	
14	Posterior layer of oblique aponeurosis	
15	Linea semilunaris	
16	Anterior layer of oblique aponeurosis	
17	Superficial inguinal lymph nodes	
18	Pubic tubercle	
19	Pyramidalis	
20	Pubic symphysis	
21	Mons pubis	
22	Inguinal ring (position of)	
23	Ilioinguinal nerve	
24	Anterior superior iliac spine	
25	Inguinal ligament	
26	Tensor fascia latae	
27	Transpyloric plane	
28	Intertubercular plane	

Abdominal viscera I – *from the front*
Structures of the internal abdominal wall – *from below*

The nine regions of the abdomen:

A   Upper central – **epigastric region**
B   Central   – **umbilical region**
C   Lower central – **pubic region**

D   Right – **hypochondrium** – left
E   Right – **lateral (flank) region** – left
F   Right – **inguinal (groin) region** – left

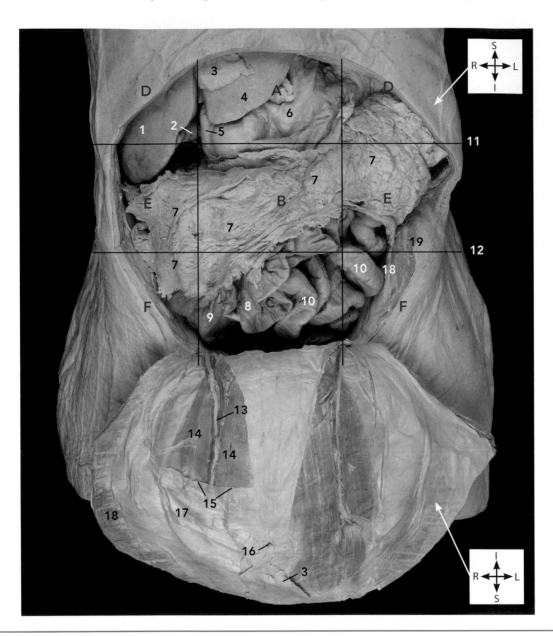

1	Right lobe of liver	9 Caecum
2	Gall bladder	10 Small intestine (coils of
3	Falciform ligament	jejunum and ileum)
4	Left lobe of liver	11 Transpyloric plane
5	Duodenum, superior (1st part)	12 Intertubercular plane plane
6	Body of stomach	13 Inferior epigastric artery and
7	Greater omentum	vein
8	Terminal part of ileum	14 Rectus abdominis

15 Arcuate line (free edge of
    posterior rectus sheath)
16 Umbilicus
17 Rectus sheath
18 Transversus abdominis
19 Internal oblique

Abdominal viscera II, with greater omentum reflected superiorly – *from the front*

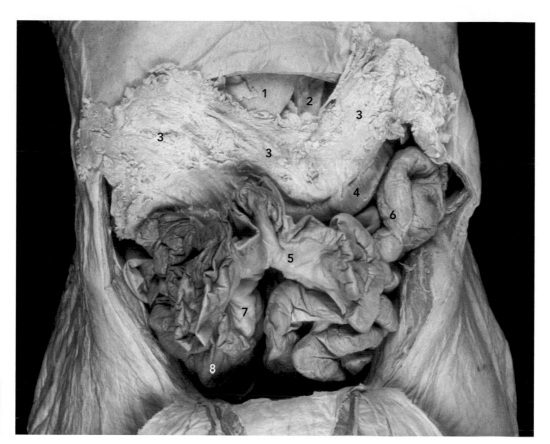

1	Left lobe of liver	4	Transverse colon	7	Ileum
2	Body of stomach	5	Mesentary	8	Caecum
3	Greater omentum	6	Jejunum		

The passage of food via the digestive alimentary tract

From the:

➤ **Mouth** – to the

➤ **Pharynx** – approximately 12–14 cm in length, extending from the base of the skull to the sixth (CVI) cervical vertebra; then into the

➤ **Oesophagus** – approximately 25 cm in length, extending from the sixth (CVI) cervical vertebra, passing through the diaphragm at the level of the tenth (TX) thoracic vertebra; to the

➤ **Stomach** – at the level of the ninth (TIX) thoracic vertebra (gastro-oesophageal junction); then through the stomachs fundus, body and pylorus; to the

➤ **Small intestine** – which is approximately 6–7 metres in total length from the pylorus of the stomach to the ileocaecal junction;

- **duodenum** – approximately 20–25 cm in total length; through the superior (1st part) 5 cm, descending (2nd part) 8–10 cm, inferior (3rd part) 10 cm, and ascending (4th part) 2.5 cm; to the
- **jejunum** – approximately 2.5 metres in length; and
- **ileum** – approximately 3.5 metres in length; to the

➤ **Large intestine** – which is approximately 1.5 metres in total length from the caecum to the anus;

- **caecum** – then from the ilocaecal junction, location of the appendix, to the
- **colon** – through its ascending, transverse, descending and sigmoid parts; to the
- **rectum** – and into
- **anal canal** – as food waste (faeces); finally exiting the
- **anus** – after travelling an overall distance from mouth to anus of approximately 9 metres.

Transverse section through the abdomen at the level of the second (LII) and third (LIII) lumbar vertebra – *from below*

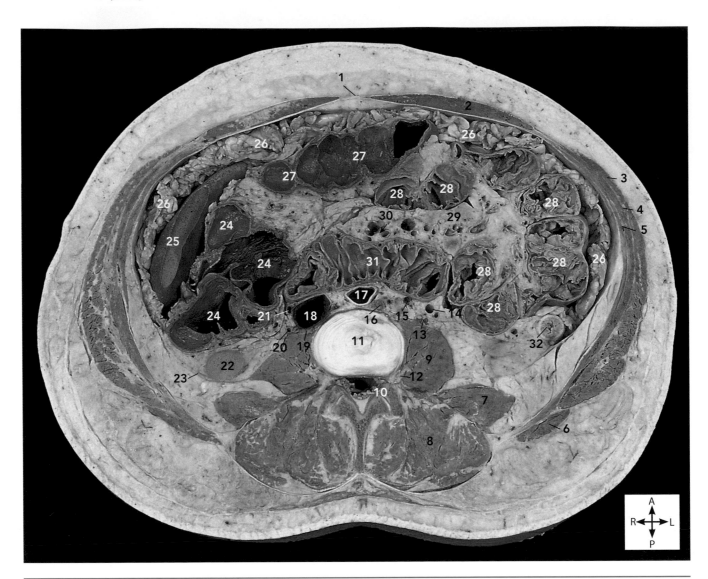

1	Linea alba	12	Root of second lumbar nerve	24	Ascending colon and right colic (hepatic) flexure
2	Rectus abdominis	13	Left ureter	25	Right lobe of liver
3	External oblique	14	Inferior mesenteric vein	26	Greater omentum
4	Internal oblique	15	Left testicular artery and vein	27	Transeverse colon
5	Transversus abdominis	16	Para-aortic lymph nodes	28	Jejunum
6	Latissimus dorsi	17	Aorta	29	Mesentary with mesenteric vessels
7	Quadratus lumborum	18	Inferior vena cava		
8	Erector spinae	19	Right sympathetic chain	30	Superior mesenteric artery and vein
9	Psoas major	20	Right ureter		
10	Cauda equina within vertebral canal	21	Right testicular artery and vein	31	Duodenum, inferior (3rd part)
11	Intervertebral disc between the second (LII) and third (LIII) lumbar vertebra	22	Lower pole of right kidney	32	Descending colon
		23	Renal fascia		

Caecum, terminal ileum (the iliocaecal junction) and vermiform appendix –
from the front

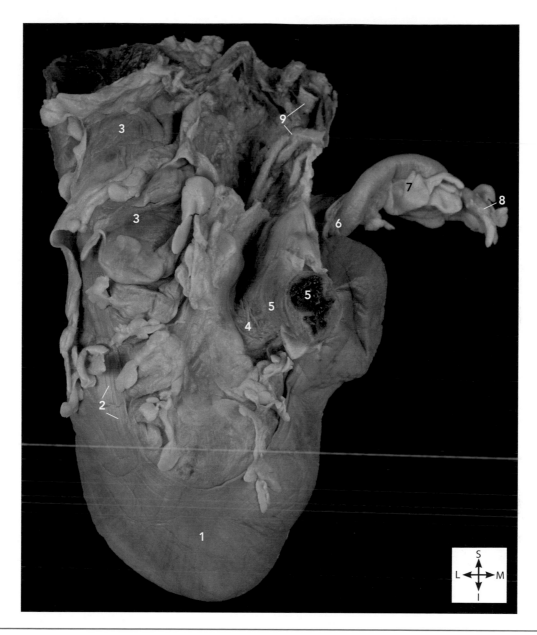

1	Caecum	6	Base
2	Anterior taenia coli (taenia libra)	7	Mesentery
3	Ascending colon	8	Tip
4	Ileocaecal junction	9	Ileocaecal artery and vein
5	Terminal ileum		

6 Base ⎤
7 Mesentery ⎬ of vermiform appendix
8 Tip ⎦

The vermiform appendix:
➤ Usually has an internal diameter of 0.5 cm.
➤ Length varies between 2 and 20 cm, with an average of 8 cm.
➤ Position is variable but consensus of research data gives:
  ● Retrocolic and retrocaecal 70%.
  ● Subcaecal and pelvic 20%.
  ● Retro-ileal and pre-ileal 5%.

Transverse section through the abdomen at the level of the first (LI) lumbar vertebra – *from below*

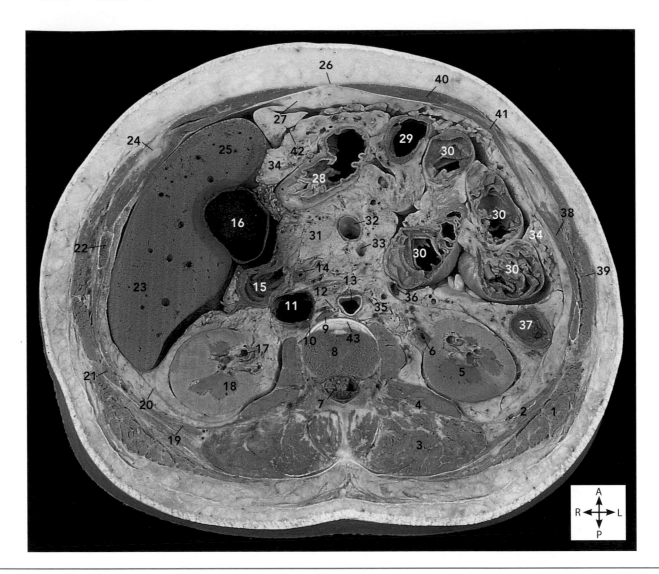

1 Latissimus dorsi	16 Gall bladder	31 Head of pancreas
2 Serratus posterior inferior	17 Commencement of right ureter	32 Superior mesenteric vein
3 Erector spinae	18 Right kidney	33 Superior mesenteric artery
4 Quadratus lumborum	19 Twelfth (XII) rib	34 Greater omentum
5 Left kidney	20 Renal fascia	35 Para-aortic lymph node
6 Left ureter	21 Eleventh (XI) rib	36 Inferior mesenteric vein
7 Cauda equina within vertebral canal	22 Tenth (X) rib	37 Descending colon
8 Body of first (LI) lumbar vertebra	23 Right lobe of liver	38 Internal oblique
9 Right crus of diaphragm	24 Ninth costal cartilage	39 External oblique
10 Right sympathetic chain	25 Left lobe of liver (medial segment)	40 Rectus abdominis
11 Inferior vena cava	26 Linea alba	41 Transverse abdominis
12 Cisterna chyli	27 Falciform ligament	42 Left lobe of liver (lateral segment)
13 Aorta	28 Antrum of stomach	43 Portion of disc between first (LI) and second (LII) lumbar vertebra
14 Common bile duct	29 Transverse colon	
15 Duodenum	30 Jejunum	

Upper abdominal viscera I, with removal of most of the small and all of the large intestine – *from the front and slightly below*

A Right subphrenic space   **C** Left subphrenic space
B Right subhepatic space   **D** Left subhepatic space

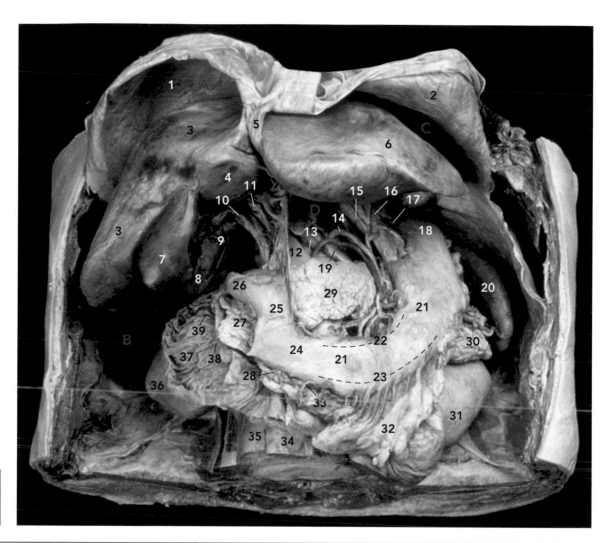

1	Right ⎤ inferior surface of the	16	Oesophagus	31	Lower pole of left kidney
2	Left ⎦ dome of diaphragm	17	Gastro-oesophageal junction	32	Greater omentum
3	Right ⎤ lobe of liver	18	Fundus of stomach	33	Right gastro-epiploic artery
4	Quadrate ⎦	19	Splenic artery	34	Aorta
5	Falciform ligament	20	Spleen	35	Inferior vena cava
6	Left lobe of liver	21	Body of stomach	36	Lower pole of right kidney
7	Fundus ⎤	22	Lesser ⎤ curvature	37	Duodenum, descending
8	Body ⎬ of gall bladder	23	Greater ⎦ of stomach		(2nd part)
9	Neck ⎦	24	Pyloric antrum	38	Major duodenal papilla with
10	Cystic duct	25	Pylorus of stomach		the common opening for the
11	Common hepatic duct	26	Duodenum, superior (1st part)		bile and main pancreatic duct
12	Portal vein	27	Head ⎤		(ampulla of Vater)
13	Common hepatic trunk	28	Uncinate process ⎬ of	39	Minor duodenal papilla with
14	Left gastric artery	29	Body ⎬ pancreas		the opening of the accessory
15	Anterior vagal trunk	30	Tail ⎦		pancreatic duct

Upper abdominal viscera II, with removal of most of the small and all of the large intestine – *from the front and slightly below*

A	Right subphrenic space	**C**	Left subphrenic space
B	Right subhepatic space	**D**	Left subhepatic space

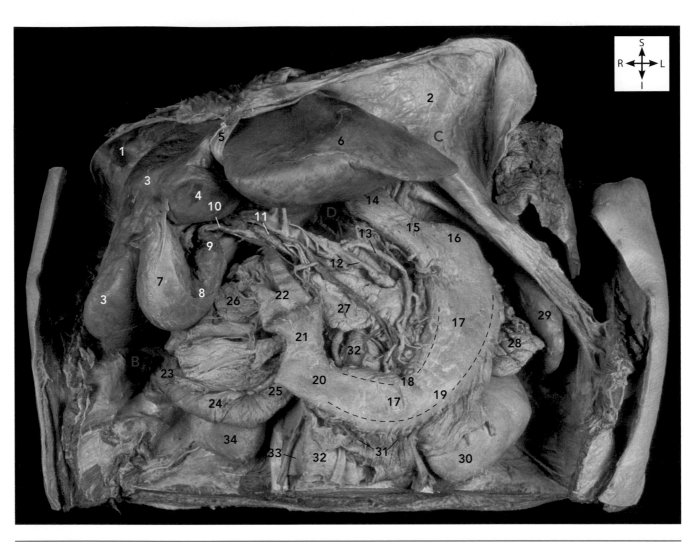

1	Right ⎤ inferior surface of the	14	Oesophagus	26	Head ⎤
2	Left ⎦ dome of diaphragm	15	Gastro-oesophageal junction	27	Body ⎥ of pancreas
3	Right ⎤ lobe of liver	16	Fundus ⎤ of stomach	28	Tail ⎦
4	Quadrate ⎦	17	Body ⎦	29	Spleen
5	Falciform ligament	18	Lesser ⎤ curvature of stomach	30	Lower pole of left kidney
6	Left lobe of liver	19	Greater ⎦	31	Gastro-epiploic vessels within greater omentum
7	Fundus ⎤	20	Pyloric antrum		
8	Body ⎥ of gall bladder	21	Pylorus of stomach	32	Aorta
9	Neck ⎦	22	Superior (1st part) ⎤	33	Inferior vena cava
10	Cystic duct	23	Descending (2nd part) ⎥ of duodenum	34	Lower pole of right kidney
11	Common hepatic duct	24	Inferior (3rd part) ⎥		
12	Splenic artery	25	Ascending (4th part) ⎦		
13	Left gastric artery				

Stomach, incised along the length of the greater curvature and opened (as a book), to expose internal structures in a coronal plane, thus views are:

A Anterior portion reflected superiorly, *from behind*   **B** Posterior portion, *from the front*

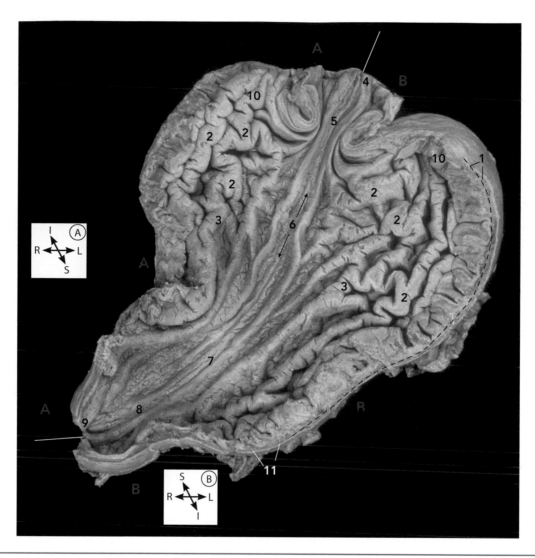

1 Greature curvature of stomach	7 Pyloric antrum
2 Folds of mucous membrane (gastric rugae)	8 Pyloric canal
3 Body of stomach	9 Pylorus (gastroduodenal junction)
4 Oesophagus at the gastro-oesophageal junction	10 Fundus of stomach
5 Cardiac part of stomach	11 Muscular coat of stomach
6 Gastric canal	

The stomach:
➤ Is shaped like the letter **J**.
➤ The gastro-oesophageal junction (upper opening into the stomach), lies to the left of the midline at the level of the ninth (TIX) thoracic vertebra.
➤ The gastroduodenal junction at the pylorus (lower opening out of the stomach), lies to the right of the midline at the level of the first (LI) lumbar vertebra.
➤ Upper border has the lesser curvature.
➤ Lower border has the greater curvature.

Liver – *from the front*

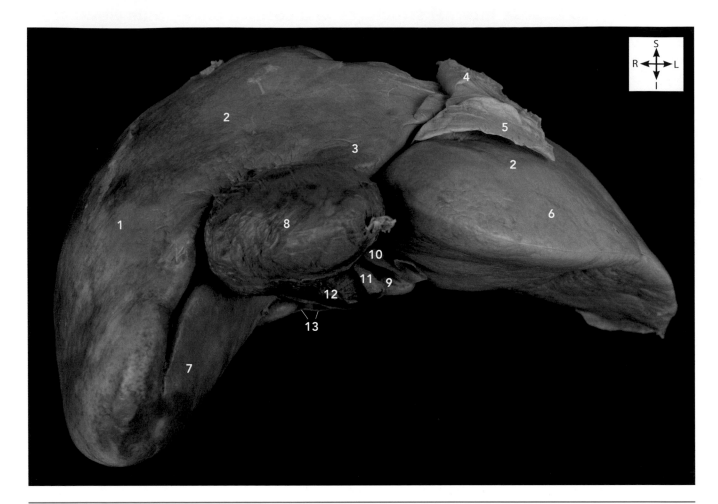

1	Right lobe	6	Left lobe	11	Common hepatic duct
2	Diaphragmatic surface	7	Colic impression	12	Portal vein
3	Quadrate lobe	8	Fundus of gall bladder	13	Inferior vena cava
4	Falciform ligament	9	Caudate lobe		
5	Ligamentum teres	10	Hepatic artery		

The morphological division of the liver into segments are:

➤ **Left part of liver**
  ● left lateral division
    – left posterior lateral segment : segment II
    – left anterior lateral segment : segment III
  ● left medial division
    – left medial segment : segment IV
➤ **Posterior part of liver**
  ● posterior segment : caudate lobe : segment I

➤ **Right part of liver**
  ● right medial division
    – anterior medial segment : segment V
    – posterior medial segment : segment VIII
  ● right lateral division
    – anterior lateral segment : segment VI
    – posterior lateral segment : segment VII

Liver – *from below*

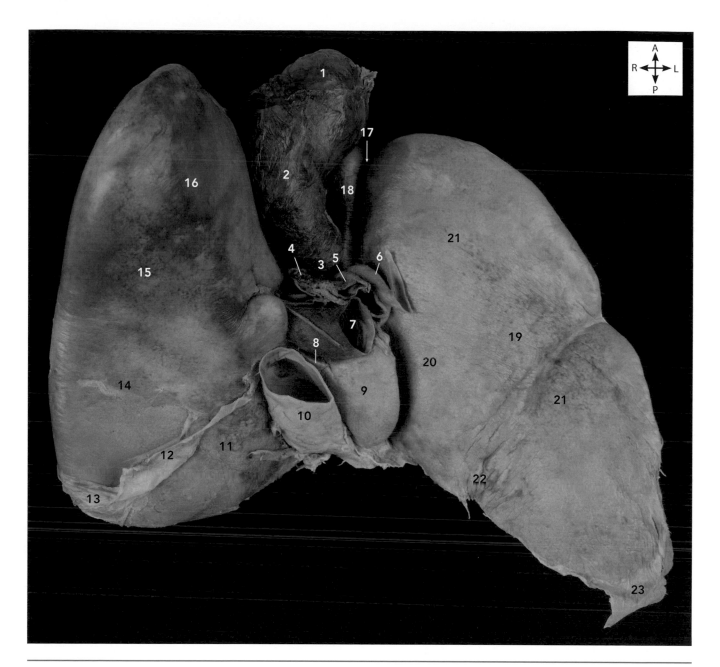

1	Fundus	9	Caudate lobe	17	Notch for ligamentum teres and falciform ligament
2	Body of gall bladder	10	Inferior vena cava	18	Quadrate lobe
3	Neck	11	Bare area	19	Gastric impression
4	Cystic duct	12	Coronary ligament	20	Omental tuberosity
5	Common hepatic duct	13	Right triangular ligament	21	Left lobe
6	Hepatic artery	14	Renal impression	22	Oesophageal groove
7	Portal vein	15	Right lobe	23	Left triangular ligament
8	Caudate process	16	Colic impression		

Pancreas – *from the front*

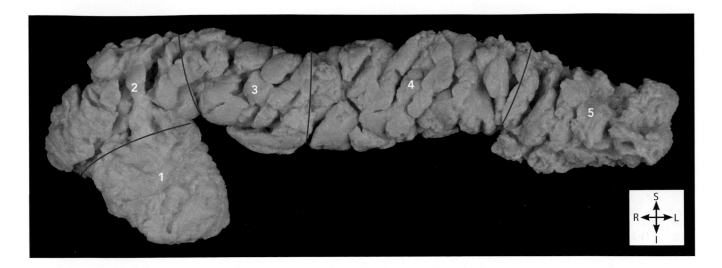

1   Uncinate process
2   Head
3   Neck
4   Body
5   Tail

The pancreas is:

➤ Normally 15 cm in length and lobulated throughout with alveoli of serous secretory cells.

➤ Has a **main duct** which runs internally throughout its length from tail to head increasing in diameter as it is joined by tributaries along its route.

➤ On exit, the main duct is joined by the **common bile duct** and both enter the main duodenal papilla (*ampulla of Vater*), which projects into the descending (2nd part) of the duodenum. It drains the tail, body, neck and upper part of the head of the pancreas.

➤ An **accessory duct** drains the lower part of the head and uncinate process, exits the pancreas and enters the minor duodenal papilla approximately 2 cm above the main duodenal papilla (ampulla of Vater).

Spleen – *A from the front; B from below*

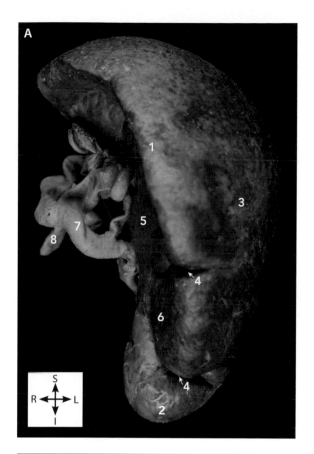

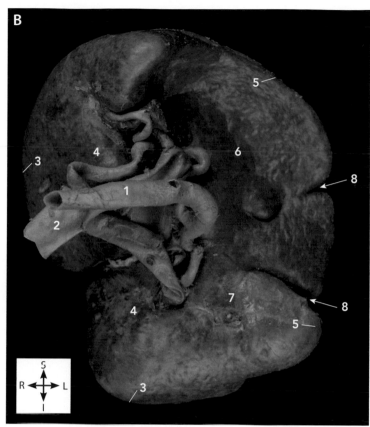

A

1 Superior border
2 Inferior border
3 Diaphragmatic surface
4 Notch
5 Gastric impression
6 Colic impression
7 Splenic artery
8 Splenic vein

B

1 Splenic artery
2 Splenic vein
3 Inferior border
4 Renal impression
5 Superior border
6 Gastric impression
7 Colic impression
8 Notch

Traditional description of the spleen:
➤ Is by the odd numbers, **1, 3, 5, 7, 9,** and **11,** which provides an *aide-memoire* to its most important average anatomical features:
- **1 × 3 × 5** inches (2.5 × 7.6 × 12.7 cm) in size.
- **7** ounces (approx. 200 g) in weight.
- Situated in the upper left of the abdomen between the **ninth** (IX) and **eleventh** (XI) ribs.

Posterior abdominal wall I – *from the front*

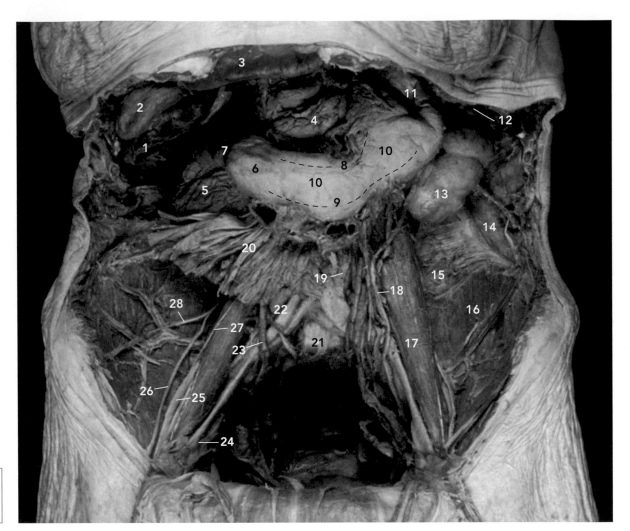

1	Right lobe of liver
2	Gall bladder
3	Left lobe of liver
4	Body ⎤ of pancreas
5	Head ⎦
6	Pylorus of stomach
7	Superior (1st part) of duodenum
8	Lesser ⎤ curvature of
9	Greater ⎦ stomach
10	Body ⎤ of stomach
11	Fundus ⎦
12	Spleen
13	Lower pole of left kidney
14	Transversus abdominis
15	Quadratus lumborum
16	Iliacus
17	Psoas major
18	Left ureter
19	Aorta
20	Right epiploic vessels in greater omentum
21	Promontary of sacrum
22	Right common iliac artery and vein
23	Right ureter
24	Right external iliac artery and vein
25	Femoral nerve
26	Lateral cutaneous nerve of thigh
27	Genitofemoral nerve
28	Ilioinguinal nerve

Posterior abdominal wall II, with stomach and duodenum reflected superiorly – *from the front*

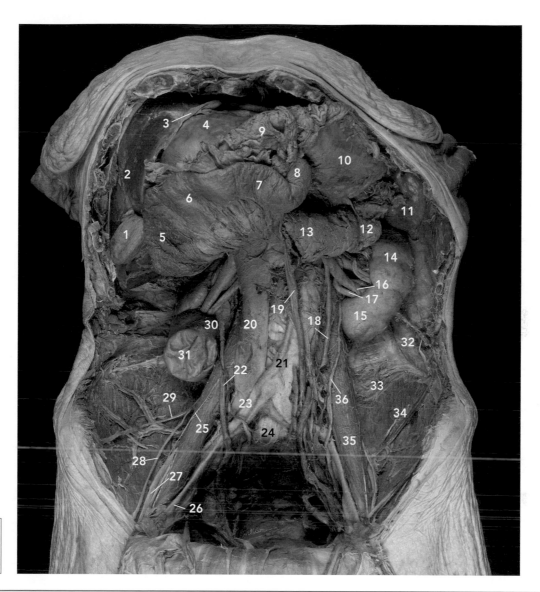

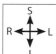

1 Gall bladder	14 Upper ⎤ pole of left kidney	27 Femoral nerve
2 Right lobe of liver	15 Lower ⎦	28 Lateral cutaneous nerve of thigh
3 Falciform ligament	16 Renal vein	29 Ilioinguanal nerve
4 Left lobe of liver	17 Renal artery	30 Lower pole of right kidney
5 Descending (2nd part) ⎤ of duodenum posterior surface	18 Gonadal vein	31 Renal cyst (deflated)
6 Inferior (3rd part)	19 Inferior mesenteric vein	32 Transversus abdominis
7 Ascending (4th part) ⎦	20 Inferior vena cava	33 Quadratus lumborum
8 Jejunum ⎤ posterior surface	21 Aorta	34 Iliacus
9 Greater omentum	22 Right ureter	35 Psoas major
10 Body of stomach ⎦	23 Right common iliac artery and vein	36 Left ureter
11 Spleen	24 Promontary of sacrum	
12 Tail ⎤ of pancreas	25 Genitofemoral nerve	
13 Body ⎦	26 Right external iliac artery and vein	

Right kidney, with adrenal gland – *from the front: A Encapsulated within perinephric fat; B With perinephric fat removed and upper part within fibrous capsule; C Isolated right adrenal gland actual size, as presented at dissection*

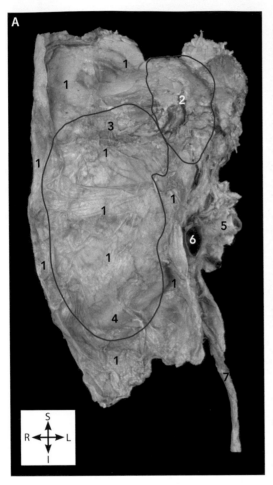

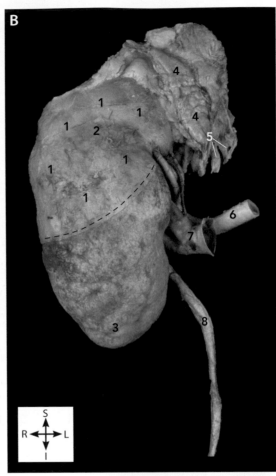

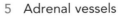

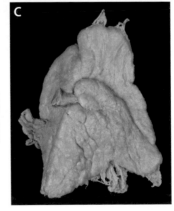

A

1 Capsule of perinephric fat (second capsule)
2 Position of adrenal gland
3 Position of upper ⎤
4 Position of lower ⎦ pole
5 Renal artery
6 Renal vein
7 Ureter

B

1 Fibrous capsule (first capsule)
2 Position of upper pole
3 Lower pole
4 Adrenal gland

5 Adrenal vessels
6 Renal artery
7 Renal vein
8 Ureter

Right kidney bisected by coronal section, posterior half – *from the front*

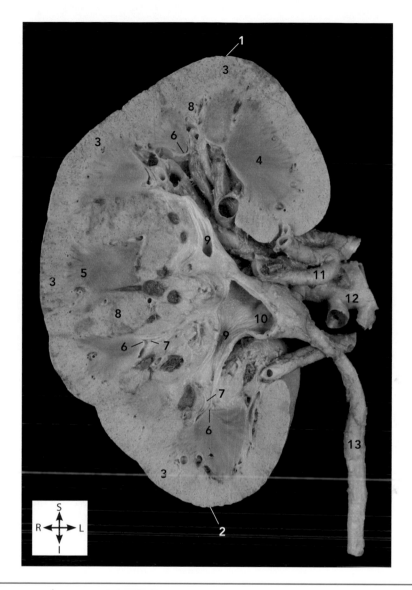

1	Upper ⎤ pole	6	Renal papilla	11	Renal artery
2	Lower ⎦	7	Minor calyx	12	Renal vein
3	Renal cortex	8	Renal column	13	Ureter
4	Medulla	9	Major calyx		
5	Medullary pyramid	10	Renal pelvis		

The kidneys:
➤ Lie retroperitoneally high up in 'gutters' on the posterior abdominal wall.
➤ The right kidney is usually 12 mm lower than the left.
➤ Are both normally 11 cm in length, 6 cm in width and 4 cm in depth.
➤ Are enveloped within three capsules, from inner to outer:
  ● **Fibrous capsule** – a very thin capsule of tissue which adheres tightly to the surface of the kidney.
  ● **Perinephric fat** – a bulky conglomeration of fat.
  ● **Renal fascia** – which is *superiorly* attached to the fascia of the diaphragm, *medially* to the aorta and inferior vena cava and *laterally* to the transversalis fascia. There is little to no attachment *inferiorly*.

Adult skeleton of pelvis, with ligaments – *from the front*

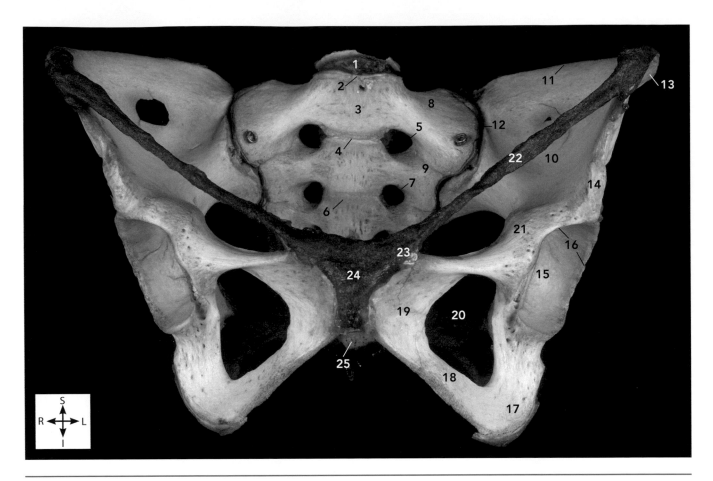

1	Intervertebral disc between fifth (LV) lumbar vertebra and sacrum	8	Upper surface of lateral part (ala)	of sacrum
2	Promontary of sacrum	9	Lateral part	
3	Sacrum (sacral verterbrae I–V)	10	Hip bone	
4	Site of fusion of first (I) and second (II) sacral vertebrae	11	Iliac crest	
5	First left pelvic sacral foramen	12	Sacro-iliac joint	
6	Site of fusion of second (II) and third (III) sacral vertebrae	13	Anterior superior	iliac spine
7	Second left sacral foramen	14	Anterior inferior	
		15	Acetabulum	
		16	Rim of acetabulum	

17	Ischial tuberosity
18	Ischiopubic ramus
19	Body of pubis
20	Obturator foramen
21	Iliopubic eminence
22	Inguinal ligament
23	Pubic tubercle
24	Pubic symphysis
25	Coccyx (coccygeal vertebrae I–IV)

The hip bone:

➤ Is formed from the fusion of three bones, the ilium, ischium and pubis.
➤ The upper part is the ilium
  ● Its upper margin being the iliac crest to the anterior or superior iliac spine at the front, and the medial surface forming the sacroiliac joint with the sacrum.
➤ The rough lower part is formed by the tuberosity of the ischium.
➤ The front part is formed by the body of the pubis.
➤ All three bones contribute to the formation of the acetabulum.
➤ Both hip bones with the sacrum and coccyx form the pelvic girdle.

Adult skeleton of pelvis, with ligaments – *from above*

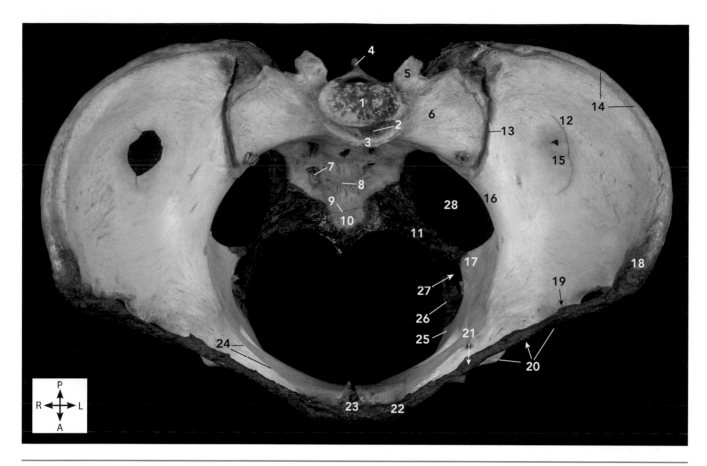

1	Body (lower portion) of fifth (LV) lumbar vertebra	
2	Intervertebral disc between fifth (LV) lumbar vertebra and sacrum	
3	Promontory of sacrum	
4	Spinous tubercle of median sacral crest	
5	Superior articular process	of sacrum
6	Lateral part (ala)	
7	Fourth right pelvic sacral foramen	
8	Site of fusion of fourth (IV) and fifth (V) sacral vertebrae	
9	Sacrococcygeal joint	
10	First (I) coccygeal vertebra	
11	Sacrospinous ligament	
12	Hip bone	
13	Sacro-iliac joint	
14	Iliac crest	
15	Iliac fossa	
16	Arcuate line	
17	Ischial spine	
18	Anterior superior	iliac spine
19	Anterior inferior	
20	Acetabulum	
21	Inguinal ligament	
22	Pubic tubercle	
23	Pubic symphysis	
24	Pectineal line	
25	Ischial tuberosity	
26	Sacrotuberous ligament	
27	Lesser	sciatic foramen
28	Greater	

A Structures within the male pelvis, left side in a paramedian sagittal section – *from the right*

B Isolated left testicle actual size as presented at dissection – *from the left*

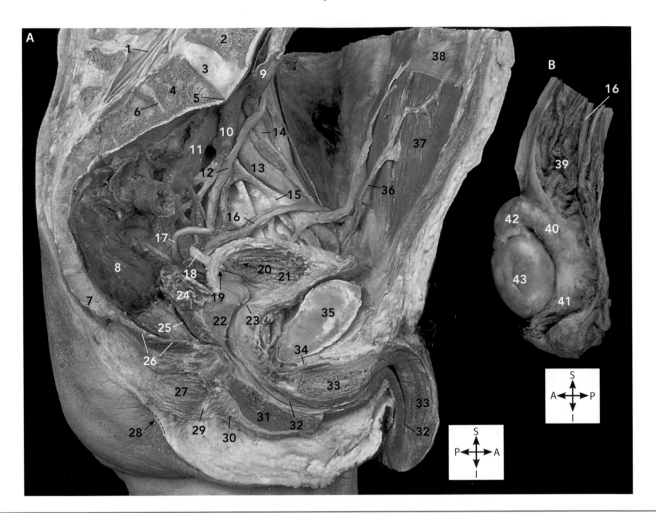

1	Cauda equina within sacral canal	
2	Body of fifth (V) lumbar vertebra	
3	Lumbosacral disc between fifth (V) lumbar vertebra and sacrum	
4	Body of first (I) sacral vertebra	
5	Promontary of sacrum	
6	Fusion between first (I) and second (II) sacral vertebrae	
7	Coccyx (coccygeal vertebrae I–IV)	
8	Rectum	
9	Common iliac artery	
10	Internal iliac artery	
11	Internal iliac vein	
12	Left ureter	

13 External iliac vein
14 External iliac artery
15 Superior vesical artery
16 Left ⎤ ductus (vas) deferens
17 Right ⎦
18 Right ureter
19 Opening of right ⎤ ureter into
20 Opening of left ⎦ bladder
21 Bladder
22 Prostate gland and prostatic part of urethra
23 Neck of bladder
24 Right seminal vesicle
25 Rectovesical pouch
26 Cut edge of levator ani
27 External anal sphincter covering anal canal
28 Anus, above arrowhead

29 Perineal body (central perineal tendon)
30 Bulbospongiosus overlying corpus spongiosum
31 Corpus spongiosum
32 Spongy part of urethra, within corpus spongiosum
33 Corpus cavernosum of penis
34 Deep dorsal vein of penis
35 Pubic symphysis
36 Inferior epigastric vessel
37 Rectus abdominis
38 Posterior wall of rectus sheath
39 Pampiniform venous plexus
40 Body ⎤
41 Tail ⎥ of epididymis
42 Head ⎦
43 Tunica albuginea around testis

A Structures within the female pelvis, left side in a paramedian sagittal section – *from the right*

B Isolated left ovary actual size as presented at dissection – *from the right*

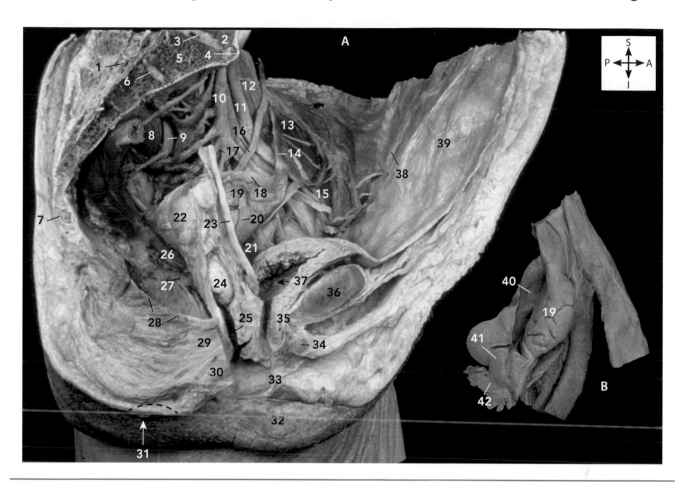

1	Sacral canal	15	Round ligament of uterus	30	Perineal body (central perineal tendon)
2	Body of fifth (V) lumbar vertebra	16	Left ureter	31	Anus, above arrowhead
3	Lumbosacral disc between fifth (V) lumbar vertebra and sacrum	17	Internal iliac vessels and branches	32	Labium majus
		18	Left broad ligament	33	Labium minus
		19	Left ovary	34	Clitoris
4	Promontary of sacrum	20	Left uterine (fallopian) tube	35	Urethra, surrounded by sphincter urethrae
5	Body of first (I) sacral vertebra	21	Vesico-uterine pouch		
6	Fusion between first (I) and second (II) sacral vertebrae	22	Body of uterus	36	Pubic symphysis
		23	Right ureter	37	Bladder, with opening of left ureter arrowed
7	Coccyx (coccygeal vertebrae I–IV)	24	Cervix of uterus		
		25	Vagina	38	Inferior epigastric vessels
8	Piriformis	26	Recto-uterine pouch (of Douglas)	39	Peritoneum overlying rectus abdominis
9	Anterior ramus of S1 nerve				
10	External iliac vein	27	Rectum	40	Posterior leaf of broad ligament
11	External iliac artery	28	Cut edge of levator ani		
12	Psoas major	29	External anal sphincter covering anal canal	41	Infundibulum of uterine tube
13	Iliacus			42	Fimbriated end of uterine tube
14	Ovarian vessels				

Male perineum, with body of penis in transverse section – *from below*

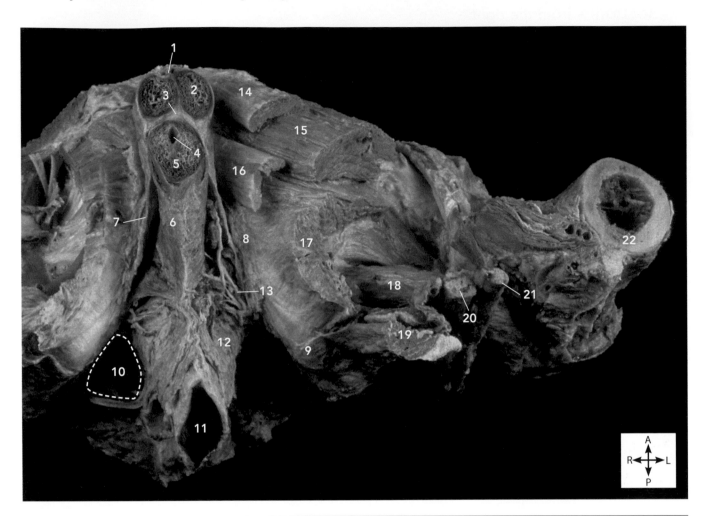

1 Dorsal artery, vein and nerve of penis	8 Ischiopubic ramus	15 Adductor brevis
2 Corpus cavernosus of penis	9 Ischial tuberosity	16 Gracilis
3 Tunica albuginea	10 Ischio-anal fossa	17 Adductor magnus
4 Urethra	11 Anal canal	18 Semitendinosus
5 Corpus spongiosum	12 Levator ani	19 Semimembrinosus
6 Bulbospongiosus	13 Internal pudendal artery and nerve	20 Sciatic nerve
7 Ischiocavernosus	14 Adductor longus	21 Gluteus maximus tendon
		22 Shaft of femur

Female perineum – *from below*

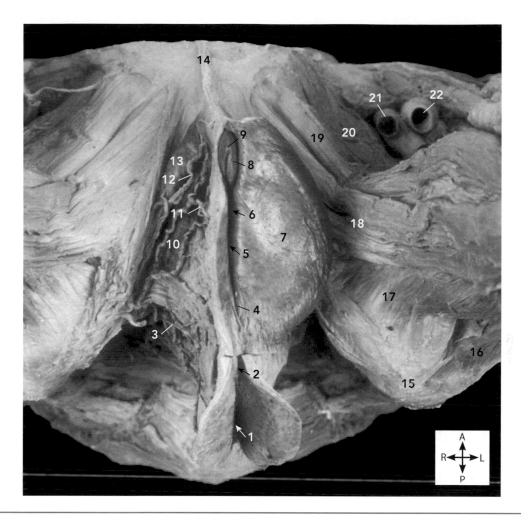

1	Anus	8	Clitoris
2	Position of perineal body	9	Prepuce of clitoris
3	Perineal branches of pudendal nerve	10	Bulb of vestibule
4	Posterior commisure	11	Posterior labial nerves
5	Vaginal opening	12	Dorsal nerve of clitoris
6	Urethral opening	13	Crura of clitoris
7	Labium majus, internal surface	14	Position of mons pubis, overlying pubic symphysis

15	Ischial tuberosity
16	Semimembranosus
17	Adductor magnus
18	Gracilis
19	Adductor longus
20	Adductor brevis
21	Femoral vein
22	Femoral artery

PART VI

Lower Limb

Adult bones of the left lower limb – *A from the front; B from behind*

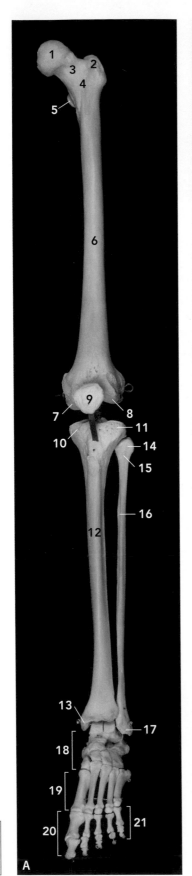

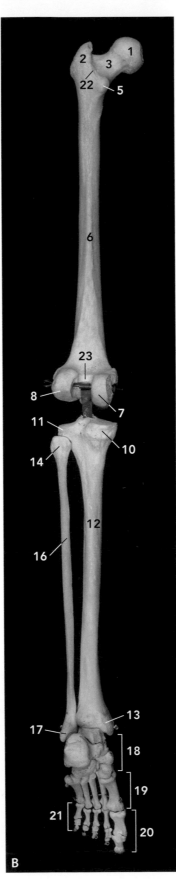

1 Head of femur
2 Greater trochanter
3 Neck of femur
4 Intertrochenteric line
5 Lesser trochanter
6 Shaft of femur
7 Medial ⎤ condyle of femur
8 Lateral ⎦
9 Patella
10 Medial ⎤ condyle of tibia
11 Lateral ⎦
12 Shaft ⎤ of tibia
13 Medial malleoulus ⎦
14 Head ⎤
15 Neck ⎥ of fibula
16 Shaft ⎥
17 Lateral malleoulus ⎦
18 Seven tarsal bones of foot
19 Five (I–V) metatarsal bones of foot
20 Two phalanges of great toe
21 Twelve phalanges of toes
22 Intertrochenteric crest of femur
23 Intercondylar fossa

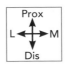

Coronal section through the left hip joint – *from the front*

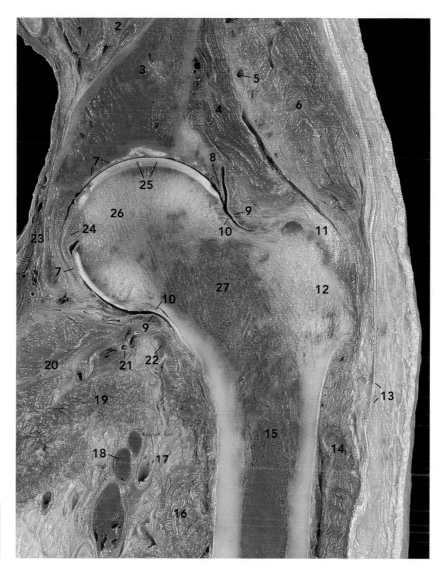

1	Psoas major	
2	Iliacus	
3	Ilium	
4	Gluteus minimus	
5	Superior gluteal artery, vein and nerve	
6	Gluteus medius	
7	Rim of acetabulum	
8	Acetabular labrum	
9	Capsule of hip joint	

10	Zona orbicularis of capsule
11	Iliofemoral ligament
12	Greater trochanter of femur
13	Iliotibial tract
14	Vastus lateralis
15	Shaft of femur
16	Vastus medialis
17	Profunda femoris artery
18	Profunda femoris vein
19	Adductor longus

20	Obturator externus
21	Medial circumflex artery and vein
22	Iliopsoas tendon
23	Obturator internus
24	Ligament of head of femur (ligamentum teres)
25	Articular cartilage
26	Head ⎫ of femur
27	Neck ⎭

The hip joint is:
➤ The largest joint in the body.
➤ Formed by the head of the femur and acetabulum of the hip bone.
➤ A synovial ball and socket joint.
➤ Capable of flexion, extension, abduction, medial and lateral rotation.
➤ Supplied by nerve fibres from the femoral, sciatic and obturator nerves.

Left gluteal region with gluteus maximus and medius severed and reflected laterally – *from behind*

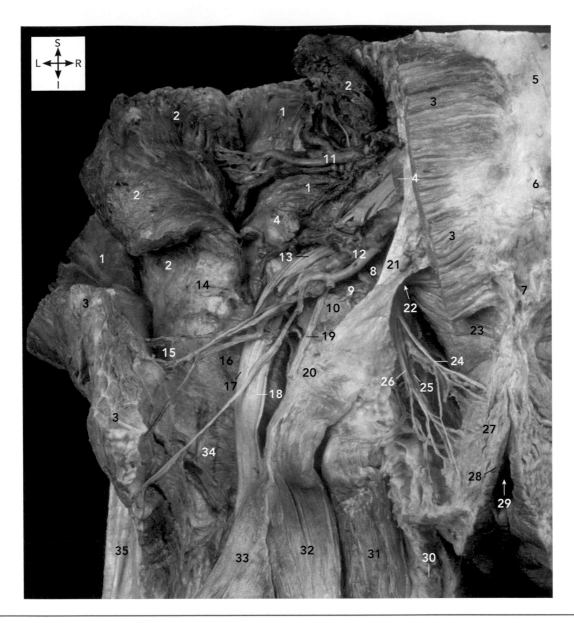

1 Gluteus minimus	13 Sciatic nerve	24 Inferior rectal artery, vein and nerve
2 Gluteus medius	14 Greater trochanter of femur	
3 Gluteus maximus	15 Vastus lateralis	25 Internal pudendal artery
4 Piriformis	16 Quadratus femoris	26 Pudendal nerve
5 Posterior layer of lumbar fascia overlying erector spinae	17 Common fibular part of sciatic nerve	27 External anal sphincter
		28 Anal margin
6 Sacrum	18 Tibial part of sciatic nerve	29 Anus
7 Coccyx	19 Posterior cutaneous femoral nerve	30 Gracilis
8 Gemellus superior		31 Adductor magnus
9 Obturator internus	20 Ischial tuberosity	32 Semitendinosus
10 Gemellus inferior	21 Sacrotuberous ligament	33 Biceps femoris (long head)
11 Superior ⎤ gluteal artery,	22 Pudendal canal	34 Upper part of adductor magnus (adductor minimus)
12 Inferior ⎦ vein and nerve	23 Levator ani	
		35 Iliotibial tract

Right gluteal region with removal of the lower outer two-thirds of gluteus maximus – *from behind*

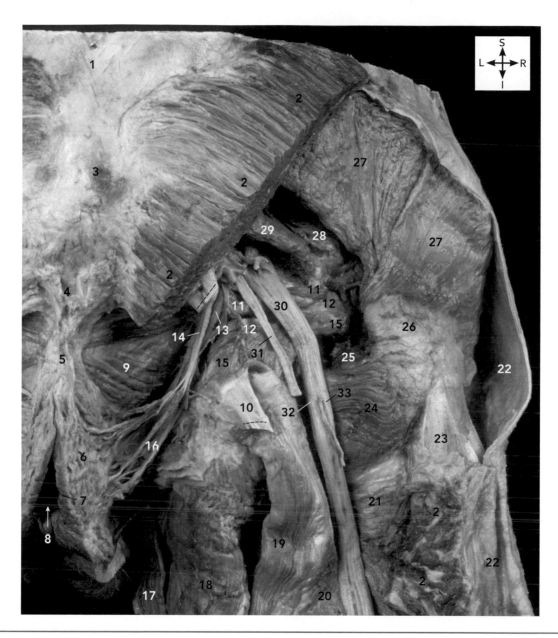

1	Posterior layer of lumbar fascia overlying erector spinae	
2	Gluteus maximus	
3	Sacrum	
4	Coccyx	
5	Anococcygeal body	
6	External anal sphincter	
7	Anal margin	
8	Anus	
9	Levator ani	
10	Sacrotuberous ligament (cut and reflected inferiorly)	
11	Gemellus superior	
12	Obturator internus	
13	Internal pudendal artery	
14	Pudendal nerve	
15	Gemellus inferior	
16	Inferior rectal artery, vein and nerve	
17	Gracilis	
18	Adductor magnus	
19	Semitendinosus	
20	Biceps femoris (long head)	
21	Upper part of adductor magnus (adductor minimus)	
22	Iliotibial tract	
23	Vastus lateralis	
24	Quadratus femoris	
25	Obturator externus	
26	Greater trochanter of femur	
27	Gluteus medius	
28	Gluteus minimus	
29	Piriformis	
30	Sciatic nerve	
31	Posterior cutaneous femoral nerve	
32	Tibial part of sciatic nerve	
33	Common fibular part of sciatic nerve	

Superficial structures of the left femoral triangle and thigh – *from the front*

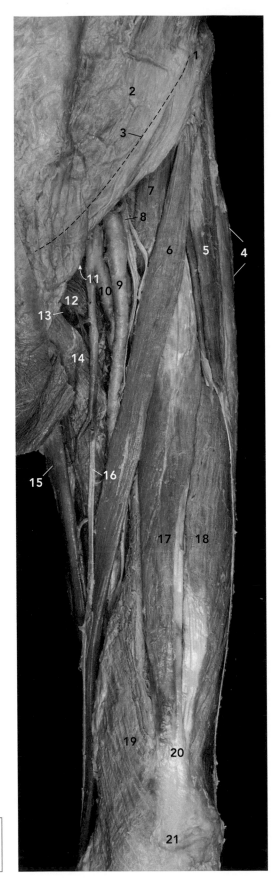

1 Anterior superior iliac spine
2 External oblique aponeurosis
3 Position of inguinal ligament
4 Iliotibial tract
5 Tensor fascia latae
6 Sartorius
7 Iliacus
8 Femoral nerve
9 Femoral artery
10 Femoral vein
11 Femoral canal
12 Pectineus
13 Adductor brevis
14 Adductor longus
15 Gracilis
16 Great saphenous vein
17 Rectus femoris
18 Vastus lateralis
19 Vastus medialis
20 Tendon of quadriceps femoris
21 Patella

The femoral triangle:
➤ Is bounded by the inguinal ligament, medial border of sartorius and medial border of adductor longus.
➤ Contains, from the lateral to medial side, the femoral nerve, artery, vein and canal.

The femoral canal:
➤ Is the most medial compartment of the femoral sheath.
➤ Is approximately 4 cm in length.
➤ Opens into the peritoneal cavity by way of the femoral ring, behind the inguinal ligament.
➤ Allows the passage of lymphatic channels from the lower limb into the pelvis.
➤ Provides space for the femoral vein to expand thus increasing venous drainage to the lower limb.

The femoral pulse:
➤ Can be palpated midway between the anterior superior iliac spine and the midline pubic symphysis (the midinguinal point or femoral point).

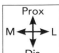

Superficial structures of the left gluteal region, thigh and popliteal fossa – *from behind*

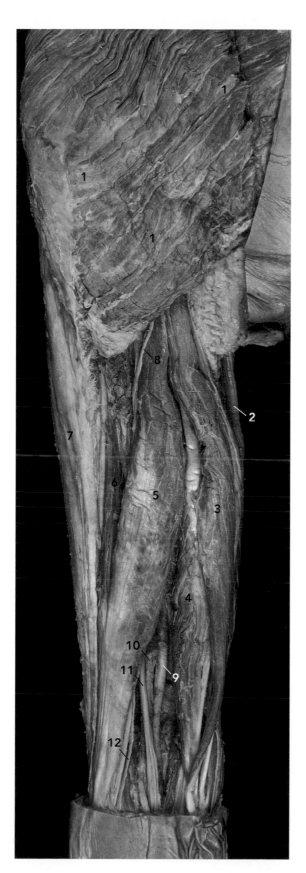

1 Gluteus maximus
2 Gracilis
3 Semimembranosus
4 Semitendinosus
5 Long head ⎤ of biceps femoris
6 Short head ⎦
7 Iliotibial tract
8 Posterior femoral cutaneous nerve
9 Popliteal artery
10 Popliteal vein
11 Tibial nerve
12 Common fibular nerve

The popliteal pulse:
➤ Requires special technique by the examiner as the poplieal artery is situated deep within the popliteal fossa surrounded by fat and tissue.
➤ With the knee flexed, both thumbs should be placed on the front of the knee; using both hands the fingers are pressed gently forwards into the middle of the fossa to locate the pulse.

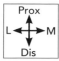

Superficial structures of the left leg – *from the front*

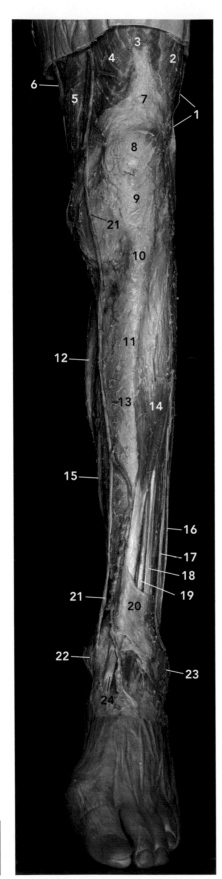

1 Cut edge of iliotibial tract
2 Vastus lateralis
3 Rectus femoris
4 Vastus medialis
5 Sartorius
6 Gracilis
7 Tendon of quadriceps femoris
8 Patella
9 Patellar ligament
10 Tuberosity ⎤ of tibia
11 Shaft ⎦
12 Medial head of gastrocnemius
13 Anterior surface of tibia
14 Tibialis anterior
15 Soleus
16 Fibularis longus
17 Superficial fibular nerve
18 Extensor digitorum longus
19 Extensor hallucis longus
20 Extensor retinaculum
21 Great saphenous vein
22 Medial malleollus of tibia
23 Lateral malleolus of fibula
24 Tendon of tibialis anterior

The patella:
➤ Is the largest sesamoid bone in the body and is situated within the quadriceps tendon.
➤ Is held at a constant distance from the upper surface of the tibia by the patellar ligament.
➤ Slides over the femoral condyles as the knee joint bends and never comes in contact with the tibia.

Prox
M ← → L
Dis

Superficial structures of the left leg and popliteal fossa – *from behind*

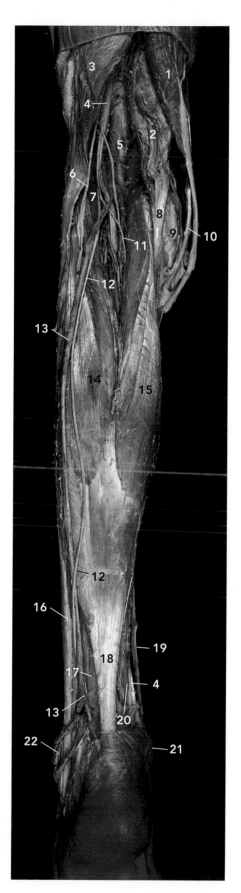

1 Semimembranosus (medially displaced)
2 Semitendinosus
3 Biceps femoris
4 Tibial nerve
5 Popliteal vein and artery
6 Common fibular nerve
7 Plantaris
8 Semitendinosus tendon
9 Position of medial condyle of tibia
10 Gracilis (tendon)
11 Muscular branches of tibial nerve
12 Sural nerve
13 Small saphenous vein
14 Gastrocnemius lateral head
15 Gastrocnemius medial head
16 Fibularis longus
17 Soleus
18 Tendo calcaneus (Achilles' tendon)
19 Great saphenous vein
20 Flexor hallucis longus
21 Medial malleolus of tibia
22 Lateral malleolus of fibula

The popliteal fossa:

➤ Is an area at the back of the knee, which is diamond in shape.
➤ Its upper boundaries are formed by:
  • On the lateral side, biceps femoris (with the common fibular nerve behind it) and on the medial side, semimembranosus (with the tendon of semitendinosus behind it).
➤ Its lower boundaries are formed by:
  • Laterally, the lateral head of gastrocnemius and plantaris and medially the medial head of gastrocnemius.
  • Superficial to deep the main structures within the fossa are the tibial nerve, popliteal vein and popliteal artery.

Sagittal section through the left knee joint – *from the left*

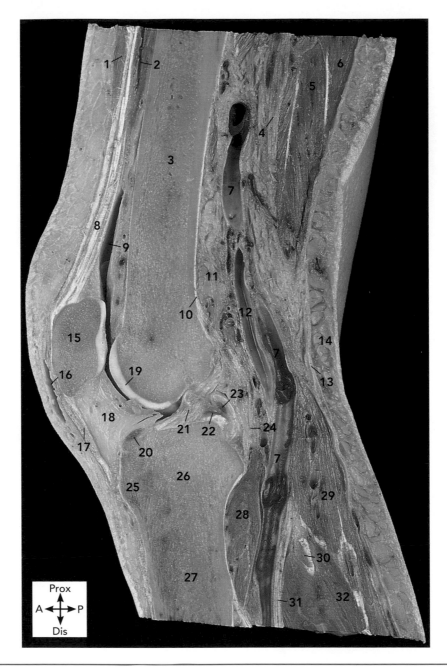

1 Rectus femoris	13 Deep fascia	23 Posterior cruciate ligament
2 Vastus intermedius	14 Superficial fascia	24 Fibrous capsule of knee joint
3 Shaft of femur	15 Patella	25 Tibial tuberosity
4 Sciatic nerve	16 Prepatellar bursa	26 Proximal end of tibia
5 Semimembranosus	17 Patellar ligament	27 Shaft of tibia
6 Semitendinosus	18 Infrapatellar pad of fat	28 Popliteus
7 Popliteal vein	19 Articular cartilage	29 Gastrocnemius
8 Tendon of quadriceps femoris	20 Anterior horn of medial meninscus	30 Tendon of plantaris
9 Suprapatellar bursa	21 Anterior cruciate ligament	31 Tibial nerve
10 Popliteal surface of femur	22 Posterior horn of medial meniscus	32 Soleus
11 Popliteal pad of fat		
12 Popliteal artery		

Adult bones of the left knee joint – *A from the front; B from behind*

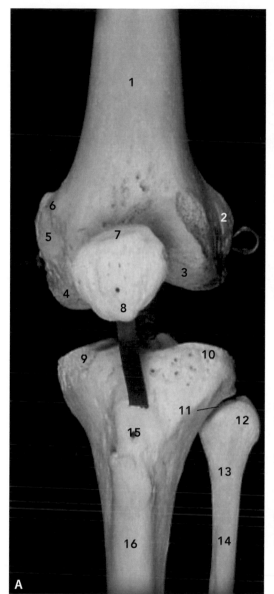

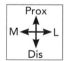

A

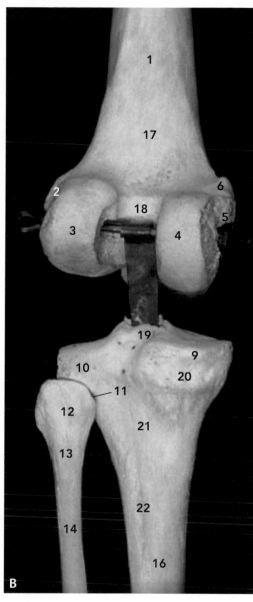

B

1	Shaft	of femur	9	Medial	condyle of tibia	17	Popliteal surface of femur
2	Lateral epicondyle		10	Lateral		18	Intercondylar fossa
3	Lateral condyle		11	Superior tibiofibular joint		19	Intercondylar eminence
4	Medial condyle		12	Head	of fibula	20	Groove for semimembranosus
5	Medial epicondyle		13	Neck		21	Popliteal surface of tibia
6	Adductor tubercle		14	Shaft		22	Soleal line
7	Base	of patella	15	Tibial tuberosity			
8	Apex		16	Shaft of tibia			

The knee joint:
➤ Is a hinge joint and the largest synovial joint in the body, formed by the unions of the two condyles of the femur and the two condyles of the tibia along with the patella, which articulates solely with the condyles of the femur.
➤ Provides movements of flexion, extension and a small degree of rotation.

Superficial structures of the left lower leg, ankle and dorsum of foot I –
from the front left and slightly above

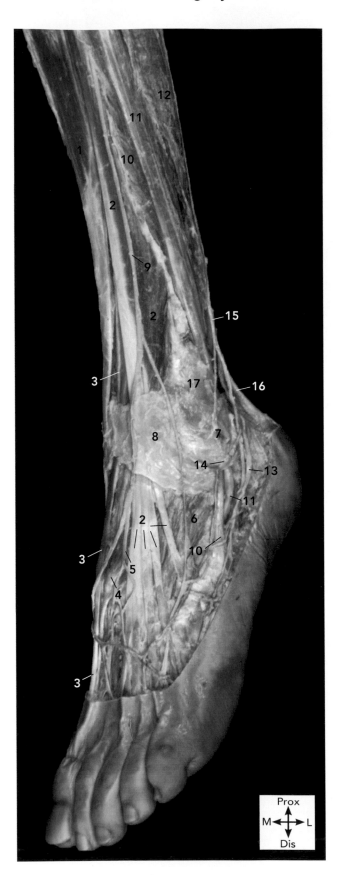

1 Tibialis anterior
2 Extensor digitorum longus
3 Extensor hallucis longus
4 Extensor hallucis brevis
5 Dorsalis pedis artery
6 Extensor digitorum brevis
7 Lateral malleolus of fibula
8 Inferior extensor retinaculum
9 Superficial fibular nerve
10 Fibularis brevis
11 Fibularis longus
12 Soleus
13 Small saphenous vein
14 Superior fibular retinaculum
15 Sural nerve
16 Tendo calcaneus (Achilles' tendon)
17 Subcutaneous area of fibula

The dorsalis pedis artery:
➤ Is absent in approximately 12% of feet.
➤ When present can be palpated along the upper part of a line from the midpoint between the lateral and medial malleolus and towards the cleft of the first toe.

Superficial structures of the left lower leg, ankle and dorsum of foot II –
from the front left and slightly above

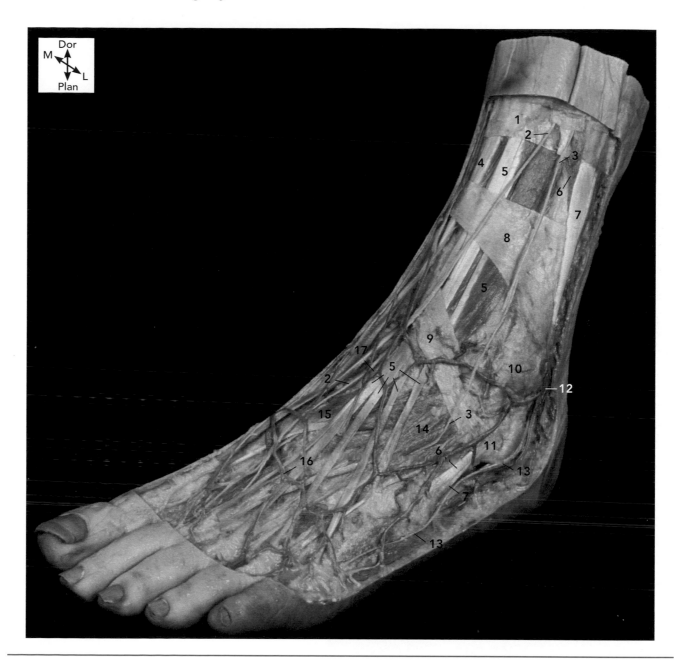

1 Deep fascia of leg	7 Fibularis longus	13 Sural nerve
2 Medial branch ⌐ of superficial	8 Superior ⌐ extensor	14 Extensor digitorum brevis
3 Lateral branch ⌐ fibular nerve	9 Inferior ⌐ retinaculum	15 Extensor hallucis brevis
4 Tibialis anterior	10 Lateral malleolus of fibula	16 Dorsal venous arch
5 Extensor digitorum longus	11 Superior fibular retinaculum	17 Dorsalis pedis artery
6 Fibularis brevis	12 Small saphenous vein	

The small saphenous vein:
➤ Runs behind the lateral malleolus of the fibula.

The great saphenous vein:
➤ Runs in front of the medial malleolus of the tibia.

Deep medial structures of the left lower leg, ankle and sole of foot I –
from the right

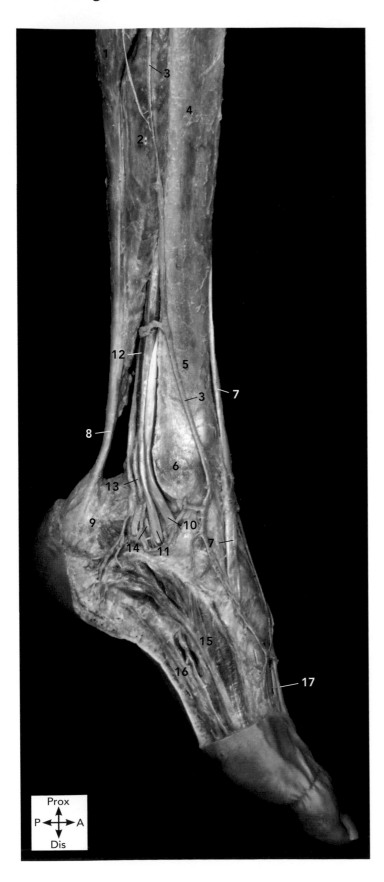

1 Gastrocnemius
2 Soleus
3 Great saphenous vein
4 Shaft ⎤
5 Medial surface ⎥ of tibia
6 Medial malleolus ⎦
7 Tibialis anterior
8 Tendo calcaneus (Achilles' tendon)
9 Medial surface of calcaneus
10 Tibialis posterior
11 Flexor digitorum longus
12 Flexor hallucis longus
13 Tibial nerve
14 Tibial artery and vein
15 Abductor hallucis
16 Plantar aponeurosis
17 Extensor hallucis longus

The tendo calcaneus (Achilles' tendon):
➤ Is the thickest tendon in the body and
   receives muscle fibres from gastrocnemius
   and soleus.
➤ Inserts into the middle of the back of the
   calcaneus.
➤ May be tested for ankle jerk, just above its
   insertion into the the calcaneus.
➤ Under exertion is prone to rupture (tear)
   usually about 2–5 cm above its insertion into
   the calcaneus, producing a palpable gap as
   fibres of the tendon 'roll-up' like a roller blind.

Deep medial structures of the left lower leg, ankle and second layer of sole of foot II – *from the right and slightly below*

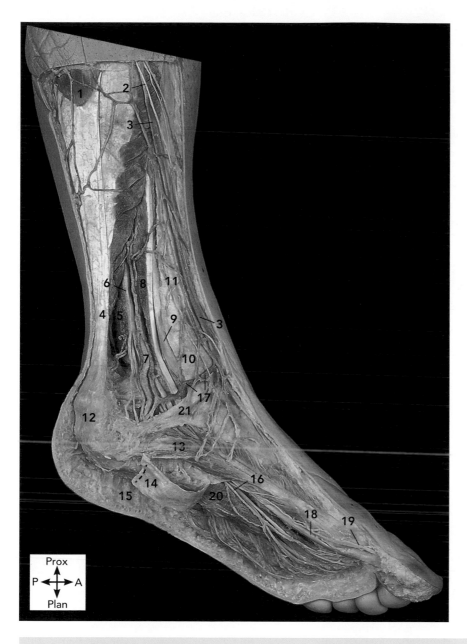

1 Gastrocnemius
2 Medial branch of superficial fibular nerve
3 Great saphenous vein
4 Tendo calcaneus (Achilles' tendon)
5 Flexor hallucis longus
6 Tibial nerve
7 Posterior tibial artery and veins
8 Flexor digitorum longus
9 Tibialis posterior
10 Medial malleolus ⎤ of tibia
11 Medial surface ⎦
12 Posterior surface of calcaneus
13 Abductor hallucis
14 Plantar aponeurosis (reflected posteriorly)
15 Dense subcutaneous fatty tissue of sole of foot
16 Medial plantar nerve
17 Dorsal venous arch
18 Tendon of flexor hallucis longus
19 Proper plantar nerve of great toe
20 Flexor digitorum brevis
21 Flexor retinaculum

The posterior tibial artery:
➤ Can be palpated behind the medial malleolus of the tibia approximately 2.5 cm in front of the medial border of the tendo calcaneus (Achilles' tendon).

The flexor retinaculum:
➤ Extends from the medial malleolus of the tibia to the side of the calcaneus and as its name quite rightly implies, keeps the flexor tendons in place.

Adult bones of the left foot – *from above*

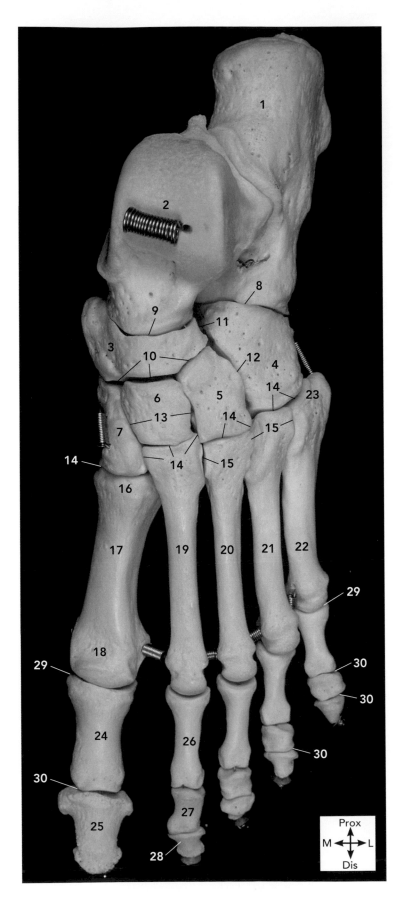

1 Calcaneus ⎤
2 Talus
3 Navicular
4 Cuboid   tarsal bones
5 Lateral cuneiform
6 Intermediate cuneiform
7 Medial cuneiform ⎦
8 Calcanocuboid joint
9 Talonavicular part of
    talocalcaneonavicular joint
10 Cuneonavicular joint
11 Cuboideonavicular joint
12 Cuneocuboid joint
13 Intercuneiform joints
14 Tarsometatarsal joints
15 Intermetatarsal joints
16 Base ⎤ of first (I)
17 Shaft ⎥ metatarsal
18 Head ⎦ bone
19 Second (II) ⎤
20 Third (III) ⎥ metatatarsal
21 Fourth (IV) ⎥ bone
22 Fifth (V) ⎦
23 Tuberosity at base of fifth (V)
    metatarsal bone
24 Proximal ⎤ phalanx of
25 Distal ⎦ great toe
26 Proximal ⎤
27 Middle ⎥ phalanx of
28 Distal ⎦ second toe
29 Metatarsophalangeal joints
30 Interphalangeal joints

Prox
M ←→ L
Dis

Adult bones of the left foot – *from below*

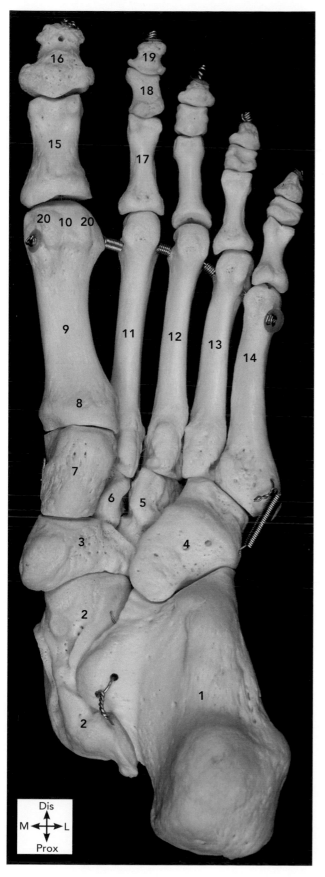

1 Calcaneus
2 Talus
3 Navicular
4 Cuboid   } tarsal bones
5 Lateral cuneiform
6 Intermediate cuneiform
7 Medial cuneiform

8 Base   ⎤ of first (I)
9 Shaft   ⎥ metatarsal
10 Head   ⎦ bone

11 Second (II)   ⎤
12 Third (III)   ⎥ metatarsal
13 Fourth (IV)   ⎥ bone
14 Fifth (V)   ⎦

15 Proximal   ⎤ phalanx of
16 Distal   ⎦ great toe

17 Proximal   ⎤
18 Middle   ⎥ phalanx of
19 Distal   ⎦ second toe

20 Grooves for sesamoid bones in flexor hallucis brevis

Coronal section through the left ankle joint and foot – *from the front*

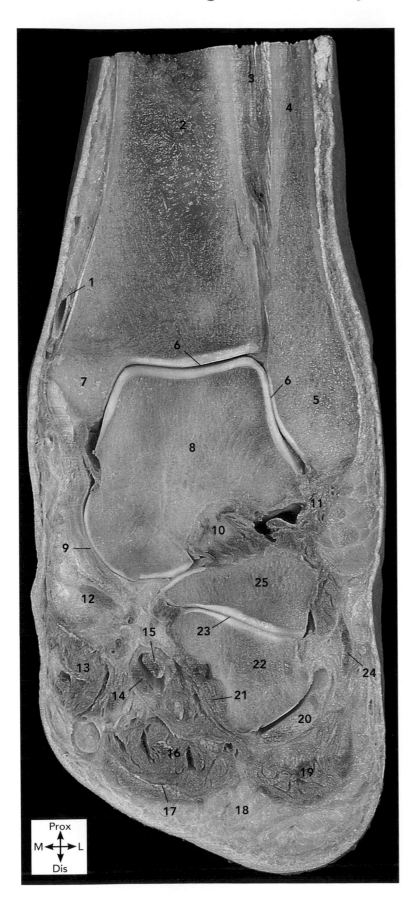

1 Small saphenous vein
2 Shaft of tibia
3 Tibialis posterior
4 Shaft of fibula
5 Lateral malleolus of fibula
6 Ankle joint
7 Medial malleolus of tibia
8 Body of talus
9 Deltoid ligament (medial collateral ligament)
10 Talocalcanean interosseous ligament
11 Lateral collateral ligament of ankle
12 Tendon of tibialis posterior
13 Abductor hallucis
14 Tendon of flexor digitorum longus
15 Tendon of flexor hallucis longus
16 Flexor digitorum brevis
17 Plantar aponeurosis
18 Dense subcutaneous fatty tissue of sole
19 Abductor digiti minimi
20 Tendon of fibularis longus
21 Quadratus plantae
22 Body of cuboid
23 Calcaneocuboid joint
24 Tendon of fibularis brevis
25 Body of calcaneus

The ankle joint:
➤ Is formed between the lower ends of the tibia and fibula and uppermost of the foot bones, the talus.

Sagittal section through the left ankle joint, foot and great toe – *from the right*

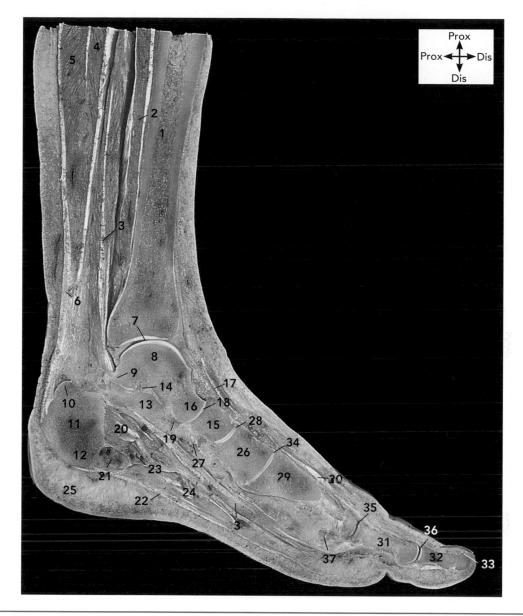

1 Shaft of tibia	14 Interosseous talocalcanean ligament	25 Dense subcutaneous fatty tissue of sole of foot
2 Flexor digitorum longus		26 Medial cuneiform
3 Tendon of flexor hallucis longus	15 Navicular	27 Tendon of tibialis posterior
4 Soleus	16 Head of talus	28 Cuneonavicular joint
5 Gastrocnemius	17 Tendon of tibialis anterior	29 First (I) metatarsal bone
6 Tendo calcaneus (Achilles' tendon)	18 Talonavicular part of talocalcaneonavicular joint	30 Extensor hallucis longus
7 Ankle joint	19 Plantar calcaneonavicular (spring) ligament	31 Proximal ⎤ phalanx of
8 Body of talus		32 Distal ⎦ great toe
9 Lateral tubercle ⎤ of talus	20 Quadratus plantae	33 Nail bed
10 Medial tubercle ⎦	21 Abductor digiti minimi	34 Cuneometatarsal joint
11 Calcaneus	22 Plantar aponeurosis	35 Metatarsophalangeal joint
12 Medial process of tuberosity of calcaneus	23 Lateral plantar artery, vein and nerve	36 Interphalangeal joint
13 Sustentaculum tali	24 Abductor hallucis	37 Sesamoid bone

Superficial structures of the left sole of foot – *from below*

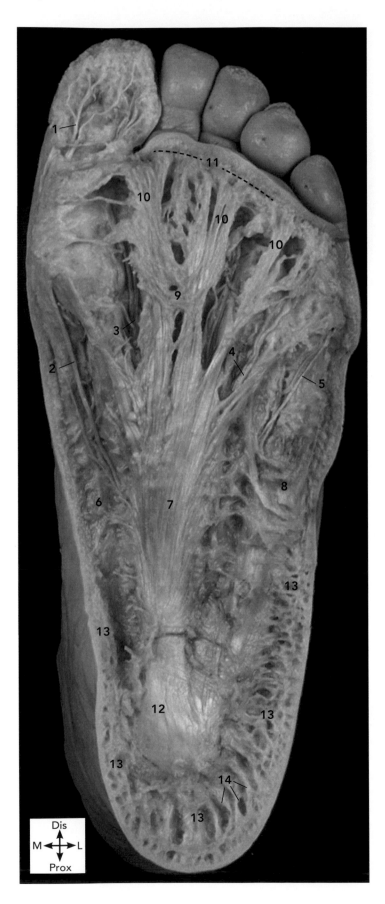

1   Medial plantar nerve, digital branches
2   Proper plantar digital nerve of great toe
3   Common plantar digital branch of medial
    plantar nerve
4   Common plantar digital branch of lateral
    plantar nerve
5   Proper plantar digital nerve of fifth toe
6   Medial part of plantar aponeurosis
    overlying abductor hallucis
7   Central part of plantar aponeurosis
    overlying flexor digitorum brevis
8   Lateral part of plantar aponeurosis
    overlying abductor digiti minimi
9   Transverse fibres of plantar aponeurosis
10 Digital slips of plantar aponeurosis
11 Superficial layer of digital band of plantar
    aponeurosis
12 Medial process of tuberosity of calcaneus
13 Dense subcutaneous fatty tissue of sole of
    foot
14 Fibrous septi forming loculations

The plantar aponeurosis:
➤ Extends from the medial and lateral tubercles
  of the calcaneus.
➤ Divides and forms five slips at the front, one
  for each toe.
➤ Fuses with the fibrous flexor sheaths and
  metatarsophalangeal joint capsules.
➤ Helps to preserve the longitudinal arches of
  the foot.

Structures of the first layer of the left sole of foot – *from below*

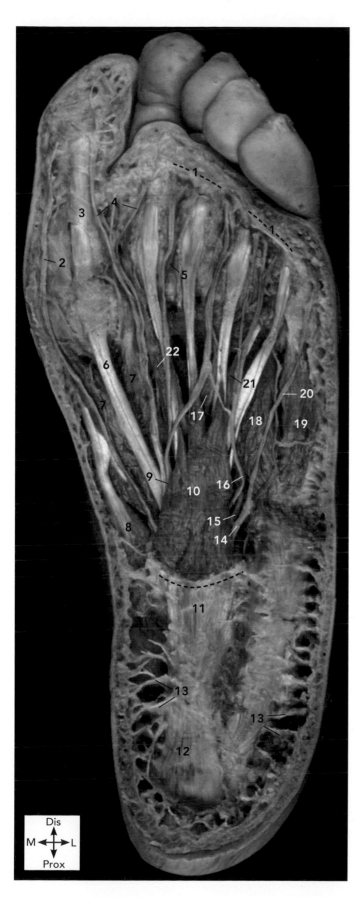

1 Superficial transverse metatarsal ligament
2 Proper plantar digital nerve of great toe
3 Fibrous flexor sheath
4 Proper plantar digital nerves of first cleft
5 Superficial digital branch of medial plantar artery
6 Flexor hallucis longus
7 Flexor hallucis brevis
8 Abductor hallucis
9 Medial plantar nerve
10 Flexor digitorum brevis
11 Central part of plantar aponeurosis
12 Medial process of tuberosity of calcaneus
13 Fibrous septi forming loculations
14 Lateral plantar nerve
15 Lateral plantar artery
16 Fourth common plantar digital nerve
17 Third lumbrical
18 Flexor digiti minimi brevis
19 Abductor digiti minimi
20 Proper plantar digital nerve of fifth toe
21 Fourth lumbrical
22 First lumbrical

The medial plantar nerve:
➤ Supplies the medial part of the sole of foot and the medial three and a half toes.

The lateral plantar nerve:
➤ Supplies the lateral part of the sole of foot and lateral one and a half toes.

Appendix

BONES OF THE BODY

The adult human skeleton is the key supporting framework of the body and normally comprises 206 bones, some single (S) and some paired (P). However, variations to this number are not uncommon, as readily seen on imaging.

CRANIUM

Parietal bone (P)
Frontal bone (S) but may be paired in cases of a frontal (metopic suture – *see* footnote on page 174)
Occipital bone (S)
Sphenoid (S)
Temporal bone (P)
Ethmoid bone (S)
Inferior nasal concha (P)
Lacrimal bone (P)
Nasal bone (P)
Vomer (S)
Maxilla (P)
Palatine bone (P)
Zygomatic bone (P)
Sutural bones (variable in number – *see* footnotes on page 174)

Stapes (P) ⎤
Incus (P) ⎬ Auditory ossicles
Malleus (P) ⎦

Mandible (S) with the Cranium, forms the Skull

NECK

Hyoid bone (S) at the level of the third (CIII) cervical vertebra

VERTEBRAL COLUMN

Cervical vertebrae (CI–CVII) – 7 in number (S)
- Atlas (CI)
- Axis (CII)   individually named vertebra
- Vertebra prominens (CVII)

Thoracic vertebrae (TI–TXII) – 12 in number (S)

Lumbar vertebrae (LI–LV) – 5 in number (S)

Sacrum (normally formed from the fusion of 5 bones – sacral vertebrae (I–V) (S)

Coccyx (normally formed by the fusion of 4 bones – coccygeal vertebrae (I–IV) (S)

THORACIC SKELETON

Ribs (I–XII) – 12 in number (P):
- True ribs (I–VII)
- False ribs (VIII–XII)
- Floating ribs (XI–XII)
- Typical ribs (III–IX)
- Atypical ribs (I, II, X, XI, XII)

Sternum (S)

UPPER LIMB

Scapula (P) ⎤
Clavicle (P) ⎦ forming pectoral (shoulder) girdle

Humerus (P) ⎤
Radius (P) ⎥ forming free part of upper limb
Ulna (P) ⎦

HAND

Scaphoid (P) ⎤
Lunate (P) ⎥
Triquetral (P) ⎥
Pisiform (P) ⎥
Trapezium (P) ⎥ carpal bones
Trapezoid (P) ⎥
Capitate (P) ⎥
Hamate (P) ⎦

Metacarpals (I–V) – 5 in number (P)

Phalanges – 14 in number (P)

Sesamoid bones (variable in number – *see* footnote, page 174)

LOWER LIMB

Hip bone (P) formed from the fusion of three bones, the ilium, ischium and pubis; and with the sacrum forms the pelvic girdle

Femur (P) ⎤
Patella (P) ⎥
Tibia (P) ⎥ forming free part of lower limb
Fibula (P) ⎦

FOOT

Talus (P) ⎤
Calcaneus (P) ⎥
Navicular (P) ⎥
Medial cuneiform (P) ⎥
Intermediate (middle) cuneiform (P) ⎥ tarsal bones
Lateral cuneiform (P) ⎥
Cuboid (P) ⎦

Metatarsals (I–V) – 5 in number (P)

Phalanges – 14 in number – (P)

Sesamoid bones (variable in number – *see* footnote, page 174)

Accessory bones (variable in number – *see* footnote, page 174)

FOOTNOTES

Frontal (metopic) suture

Frontal (metopic) suture of the frontal bone results in the adult when the two fetal frontal bones fail to fuse completely and ossify undetectably at the frontal metopic suture, thus resulting in a persisting (visible) anterior mid-line sutural division. Its occurrence has been recorded as 0–7.4% in individuals of various ethnic groups.[1] (Berry 1975).

Sutural (wormian) bones

Sutural (Wormian) bones arise from separate centres of ossification occurring at fontenelles and within or adjacent to cranial sutures of the developing fetal skull. They are most frequently located in the posterior lateral lambdoid suture and are usually irregular in shape and size. They may occur as a large single bone, which is often referred to as an 'Inca' bone, or quite commonly, as multiple small bones. The latter are associated with hydrocephalic skulls and thought to be a result of rapid cranial expansion.

Sesamoid bones

Sesamoid bones occur in both the hand and the foot. They vary in shape and size but are generally ovoid and only a few millimetres in diameter. Sesamoid bones are not always ossified completely and may consist of fibrous tissue or cartilage. The patella is the largest sesamoid bone in the body, situated over the bony joint of the knee and strung between (and within) two tendons. The patella clearly displays the theoretical function of a sesamoid, which is thought to protect tendons from wear by altering the angle of their insertion into bone and thus provide greater mechanical advantage to the joint.

In the hand (thumb): a pair of sesamoid bones are normally found on the palmar (medial) surface of the head of the first (I) metacarpal bone within the tendons of adductor pollicis (on the ulnar side) and flexor pollicis brevis (on the radial side).

In the foot (great toe): a pair of sesamoid bones are normally found in grooves, one lateral and one medial, on the plantar surface of the head of the first (I) metatarsal bone within the tendons of flexor hallucis brevis.

Accessory or supernumerary bones

Bones of the body gradually begin to form during early development phases of the fetus by initial formation of central areas of ossification within the cartilaginous and membranous skeleton. These ossification centres continue to grow and unite and eventually form solid adult bones, some during late childhood and some as late as early adulthood. Occasionally centres of ossification fail to fuse completely, often at the ends of forming bones and so create separate accessory or supernumerary bones.

The foot is a particularly common place to find accessory bones and in defined locations. The majority are directly associated with a particular bones, as their name implies.

- **Dorsum of foot:**
  - Os intercuneiforme
  - Os talonaviculare dorsal
  - Os calcaneus secondaris
  - Os intermetatarsal I
- **Posterior part of foot:**
  - Os trigonum
- **Lateral part of foot:**
  - Os calcaneus secondaris
  - Os vesalianum pedis
- **Medial part of foot:**
  - Os tibiale externum (Os naviculare accessorium)
  - Os sustentaculi
- **Plantar aspect (sole) of foot:**
  - Pars peronea metatarsalis I
  - Os cuboides secondarius

MUSCLES OF THE BODY

There are approximately 640 muscles (320 pairs) in the normal adult human body, the more important muscles are described with a brief synopsis of their attachments (**At**), actions (**Ac**) and nerve supply (**Ne**). A few smaller or less important muscles are mentioned in name only since for most medical students detailed knowledge of them is not required being more for the specialist.

HEAD AND NECK

Scalp and facial muscles

Occipitofrontalis

> At: From the highest nuchal line to the epicranial aponeurosis (occipital belly) and from the aponeurosis to blend with the orbicularis oculi and skin (frontal belly, which has no bony attachment).
> Ac: Movement of the scalp and wrinkling of the forehead.
> Ne: Facial nerve.

Orbicularis oculi

> At: From the frontal process of the maxilla and anterior lacrimal crest of the lacrimal bone (orbital part) and medial palpebral ligament (palpebral part), forming concentric loops in the eyelids and round the orbital margins.
> Ac: Closure and 'screwing up' of the eyelids.
> Ne: Facial nerve.

Orbicularis oris

> At: Circular fibres within the lips, blending at sides with the buccinators.
> Ac: Closure of the lips.
> Ne: Facial nerve.

Buccinator

> At: From pterygomandibular raphe and maxilla and mandible opposite the three molar teeth, forward to blend with the orbicularis oris.
> Ac: Compression of the cheek against gums, keeping food in the mouth cavity.
> Ne: Facial nerve.

Procerus

Nasalis

Corrugator supercilii

Levator palpebrae superioris – see page 180, under **Extrinsic muscles of the eyeball**

Levator labii superioris

Levator labii superioris alaeque nasi

Zygomaticus major

Zygomaticus minor

Levator anguli oris

Depressor anguli oris

Mentalis

Risorius

Masticatory muscles

Lateral pterygoid

At: From the infratemporal surface of the greater wing of sphenoid (upper head) and lateral surface of the lateral pterygoid plate (lower head) to the neck of the mandible and capsule and disc of the temporomandibular joint.

Ac: Opening the mouth wide and assisting side-to-side chewing movements.

Ne: Mandibular nerve.

Medial pterygoid

At: From the medial surface of the lateral pterygoid plate, pyramidal process of palatine and tuberosity of maxilla to the lower part of the medial surface of the ramus and angle of the mandible.

Ac: Closure of the mouth and assisting side-to-side chewing movements.

Ne: Mandibular nerve.

Temporalis

At: From the temporal fossa and overlying fascia to the coronoid process and anterior margin of the ramus of the mandible.

Ac: Closure of the mouth.

Ne: Mandibular nerve.

Masseter

At: From the zygomatic arch to the outer surface of the ramus of the mandible.

Ac: Closure of the mouth.

Ne: Mandibular nerve.

Neck

Platysma

At: Fascia over the upper pectoralis major to the lower part of the body of the mandible and adjacent skin and facial muscles.

Ac: Wrinkling the skin of the neck.

Ne: Facial nerve.

Sternocleidomastoid

At: From the upper front part of the manubrium of the sternum (sternal head) and medial third of the clavicle (clavicular head) to the mastoid process of the temporal bone and adjoining occipital bone.

Ac: Tilting the face and head upwards and to the opposite side.

Ne: Accessory nerve (spinal part).

Trapezius – see page 181, under **Pectoral girdle muscles**

Scalenus anterior

At: From the transverse processes of vertebrae (CIII–VI) to scalene tubercle of the first rib (I).

Ac: Elevation of the first rib.

Ne: Anterior rami of C4–6.

Scalenus medius

At: From the transverse processes of axis (CII) and vertebrae (CIII–VII) to upper surface of the first rib between the scalene tubercle and groove for the subclavian artery.
Ac: Elevation of the first rib.
Ne: Anterior rami of C5–8.

Longus colli
Longus capitis

Suboccipital muscles
Rectus capitis anterior
Rectus capitis lateralis

Suprahyoid muscles
Digastric

At: Digastric groove on the medial side of the mastoid process (posterior belly) and digastric fossa on the inner surface of the mandible (anterior belly); intermediate tendon held by a fascial sling to the lesser horn of the hyoid bone.
Ac: Depression of the mandible and elevation of the hyoid bone.
Ne: Facial nerve (posterior belly) and nerve to mylohyoid (anterior belly).

Stylohyoid

At: From back of the upper part of the styloid process to the base of the greater horn of the hyoid bone.
Ac: Elevation of the hyoid bone.
Ne: Facial nerve.

Mylohyoid

At: From the mylohyoid line of the mandible to the anterior surface of the body of the hyoid bone and midline raphe.
Ac: Elevation of the tongue and hyoid bone.
Ne: Own nerve from the inferior alveolar nerve.

Geniohyoid

At: From the inferior mental spine of the mandible to the upper border of the body of the hyoid bone.
Ac: Elevation of the hyoid bone.
Ne: Hypoglossal nerve, by C1 fibres.

Infrahyoid muscles
Sternohyoid

At: From back of the manubrium to the lower border of the hyoid bone.
Ac: Depression of the hyoid bone and larynx.
Ne: Ansa cervicalis, C1–3.

Sternothyroid

At: From back of the manubrium below the sternohyoid to the oblique line of the thyroid cartilage.
Ac: Depression of the larynx.
Ne: Ansa cervicalis, C2, 3.

Omohyoid

At: From the hyoid bone lateral to the sternohyoid (superior belly) and transverse scapular ligament and upper border of scapula (inferior belly); intermediate tendon bound by a fascial sling above the clavicle.
Ac: Depression of the hyoid bone and larynx.
Ne: Ansa cervicalis, C1–3.

Thyrohyoid

At: From greater horn of the hyoid bone to the oblique line of the thyroid cartilage above the sternothyroid.
Ac: Depression of the hyoid bone or elevation of the larynx.
Ne: Hypoglossal nerve, by C1 fibres.

Pharyngeal muscles

Superior constrictor

At: From the medial pterygoid plate and hamulus, pterygomandibular raphe and adjacent mandible to the pharyngeal raphe and tubercle.
Ac: Peristaltic action in swallowing.
Ne: Pharyngeal plexus.

Middle constrictor

At: From the stylohyoid ligament and lesser and greater horns of the hyoid bone to the pharyngeal raphe.
Ac: Peristaltic action in swallowing.
Ne: Pharyngeal plexus.

Inferior constrictor

At: From the thyroid and cricoid cartilages to the pharyngeal raphe.
Ac: Peristaltic action in swallowing and elevation of the larynx.
Ne: Pharyngeal plexus.

Stylopharyngeus

At: From the upper part of the styloid process to the back of the thyroid lamina.
Ac: Elevation of the larynx.
Ne: Glossopharyngeal nerve.

Palatopharyngeus

At: From the hard palate and palatine aponeurosis to the back of the thyroid lamina.
Ac: Elevation of the larynx and sphincteric action on the oropharyngeal isthmus.
Ne: Pharyngeal plexus.

Salpingopharyngeus

At: From the cartilage of the auditory tube, passing down to blend with the constrictors.
Ac: Opening the auditory tube.
Ne: Pharyngeal plexus.

Muscles of the soft palate and fauces

Palatopharyngeus – see above

Palatoglossus

At: From the palatine aponeurosis to blend with the styloglossus.
Ac: Elevation of the tongue.
Ne: Hypoglossal nerve.

Tensor veli palatini

At: From the scaphoid fossa, lateral lamina of the auditory tube and spine of the sphenoid to the palatine aponeurosis.
Ac: Stabilization of the palatine aponeurosis and opening of the auditory tube.
Ne: Nerve to the medial pterygoid (mandibular nerve).

Levator veli palatini

At: From the apex of the petrous temporal bone to the palatine aponeurosis.
Ac: Elevation of the palate.
Ne: Pharyngeal plexus.

Musculus uvulae

At: From the posterior nasal spine to the palatine aponeurosis.
Ac: Elevation of the uvula.
Ne: Pharyngeal plexus.

Muscles of the tongue

Genioglossus

At: From the superior mental spine to the body of the hyoid bone.
Ac: Protrusion and depression of the tongue.
Ne: Hypoglossal nerve.

Hyoglossus

At: From the body and greater horn of the hyoid bone to the side of the tongue.
Ac: Depression of the tongue.
Ne: Hypoglossal nerve

Styloglossus

At: From the tip of the styloid process and stylohyoid ligament to the back and side of the tongue.
Ac: Elevation and retraction of the tongue.
Ne: Hypoglossal nerve.

Palatoglossus – see page 178, under Muscles of the soft palate and fauces

Intrinsic muscles

At: Superior and inferior longitudinal, transverse and vertical, with no external attachment.
Ac: Alteration of tongue shape.
Ne: Hypoglossal nerve.

Laryngeal muscles

Cricothyroid

At: From the anterolateral part of the cricoid cartilage to the inferior horn and lower border of the lamina of the thyroid cartilage.
Ac: Tensor of vocal folds.
Ne: External laryngeal nerve.

Posterior crico-arytenoid

At: From the back of the lamina of the cricoid cartilage to the muscular process of the arytenoid cartilage.
Ac: Abduction of vocal folds.
Ne: Recurrent laryngeal nerve.

Lateral crico-arytenoid

At: From the upper border of the cricoid cartilage to the muscular process of the arytenoid cartilage.
Ac: Adduction of vocal folds.
Ne: Recurrent laryngeal nerve.

Transverse arytenoid

At: Between the backs of both arytenoid cartilages.
Ac: Adduction of the vocal folds.
Ne: Recurrent laryngeal nerve.

Oblique arytenoid

At: From the muscular process of one arytenoid cartilage to the apex of the opposite arytenoid cartilage.
Ac: Adduction of the ary-epiglottic fold.
Ne: Recurrent laryngeal nerve.

Thyro-arytenoid

At: From the lower part of front of the lamina of the thyroid cartilage and cricothyroid ligament to the side of the arytenoid cartilage. Lower fibres from the vocalis muscle; uppermost fibres run to the epiglottic cartilage as the thyro-epiglottic muscle.
Ac: Relaxation and adduction of the vocal folds.
Ne: Recurrent laryngeal nerve.

Extrinsic muscles of the eyeball

Levator palpebrae superioris

At: From the inferior surface of the lesser wing of the sphenoid to the tarsus and skin of the upper eyelid.
Ac: Elevation of the upper eyelid.
Ne: Oculomotor nerve and sympathetic fibres.

Superior rectus

At: From the upper part of the tendinous ring and sheath of the optic nerve to the upper part of the sclera in front of the coronal equator.
Ac: Elevation and medial rotation of the eye.
Ne: Oculomotor nerve.

Inferior rectus

At: From the lower part of the tendinous ring to the inferior surface of the sclera in front of the coronal equator.
Ac: Depression and medial rotation of the eye.
Ne: Oculomotor nerve.

Medial rectus

At: From the medial part of the tendinous ring and sheath of the optic nerve to the medial surface of the sclera in front of the coronal equator.
Ac: Medial rotation of the eye.
Ne: Oculomotor nerve.

Lateral rectus

At: From the lateral part of the tendinous ring bridging the superior orbital fissure to the lateral surface of the sclera in front of the coronal equator.
Ac: Lateral rotation of the eye.
Ne: Abducent nerve.

Superior oblique

At: From the body of the sphenoid above and medial to the optic canal and medial rectus to the upper outer quadrant of the sclera behind the coronal equator.

Ac: Depression and lateral rotation of the eye.

Ne: Trochlear nerve.

Inferior oblique

At: From the orbital surface of the maxilla lateral to the nasolacrimal groove to the lower outer quadrant of the sclera behind the coronal equator.

Ac: Elevation and lateral rotation of the eye.

Ne: Oculomotor nerve.

UPPER LIMB

Shoulder muscles

Deltoid

At: From the lateral third of the clavicle, acromion and lower border of the spine of scapula to the deltoid tuberosity of the humerus.

Ac: Abduction, flexion and medial rotation (anterior fibres) and extension and lateral rotation (posterior fibres) of the arm.

Ne: Axillary nerve, C5, 6.

Supraspinatus

At: Supraspinous fossa of the scapula to the upper facet of the greater tubercle of the humerus.

Ac: Abduction of the arm and stabilization of the shoulder joint.

Ne: Suprascapular nerve, C5, 6.

Infraspinatus

At: Infraspinous fossa of the scapula to the middle facet of the greater tubercle of the humerus.

Ac: Lateral rotation of the arm and stabilization of the shoulder joint.

Ne: Suprascapular nerve, C5, 6.

Teres minor

At: Back of the inferior angle of the scapula to the lower facet of the greater tubercle of the humerus.

Ac: Lateral rotation of the arm and stabilization of the shoulder joint.

Ne: Axillary nerve, C5, 6.

Teres major

At: Back of the inferior angle of the scapula to the medial lip of the intertubercular groove of the humerus.

Ac: Medial rotation, adduction and extension of the arm.

Ne: Lower scapular nerve, C5, 6.

Subscapularis

At: Subscapular fossa of the scapula to the lesser tubercle of the humerus.

Ac: Medial rotation of the arm and stabilization of the shoulder joint.

Ne: Upper and lower subscapular nerves, C5, 6

Pectoral girdle muscles

Muscles connecting limb to the vertebral column

Trapezius

At: From the occipital bone, ligamentum nuchae and spines of (CVII–TXII) vertebrae to the lateral third of the clavicle, acromion and upper lip of the spine of the scapula.

Ac: Upper fibres: elevation and rotation of the scapula; lower fibres: depression of the scapula; middle fibres: retraction of the scapula.
Ne: Accessory nerve, spinal part, C1–6.

Latissimus dorsi

At: From the spines of (TVII–XII) and all L vertebrae and lumbar fascia to the floor of the intertubercular groove of the humerus.
Ac: Adduction and medial rotation of the arm, and extension (if flexed).
Ne: Thoracodorsal nerve, C6–8.

Levator scapulae

At: From the transverse processes of (CI–IV) vertebrae to the vertebral border of the scapula from the base of the spine to superior angle.
Ac: Elevation of scapula.
Ne: Nerves from C3, 4.

Rhomboid minor

At: From the spines of (CVII–TI) vertebrae to the vertebral border of the scapula from the base of the spine to inferior angle.
Ac: Retraction and elevation of the scapula.
Ne: Dorsal scapular nerve, C4, 5.

Rhomboid major

At: From the spines of (TII–V) vertebrae to the vertebral border of the scapula from the base of the spine to inferior angle.
Ac: Retraction and elevation of the scapula.
Ne: Dorsal scapular nerve, C4, 5.

Muscles connecting limb to thoracic wall

Pectoralis major

At: From the lateral half of the clavicle (clavicular head), body of sternum (sternocostal head) and costal cartilages 1–7 to the lateral lip of the intertubercular groove of the humerus.
Ac: Adduction, medial rotation, flexion (clavicular head) and extension (sternocostal head) of the arm.
Ne: Medial and lateral pectoral nerves, C5–8, T1.

Pectoralis minor

At: From ribs 3–5 near costal cartilages to the coracoid process of the scapula.
Ac: Rotation and depression of the scapula.
Ne: Medial and lateral pectoral nerves, C6–8.

Serratus anterior

At: From the upper 8 ribs to the vertebral border of the scapula.
Ac: Protraction and rotation of the scapula.
Ne: Long thoracic nerve, C5–7.

Subclavius

At: From rib 1 and the costal cartilage to the groove on the clavicle.
Ac: Stabilization of the clavicle.
Ne: Own nerve, C5, 6.

Upper arm muscles

Biceps brachii

At: From the supraglenoid tubercle of the scapula (long head) and the coracoid process of the scapula (short head) to the tuberosity of the radius.

Ac: Flexion and supination of the forearm.
Ne: Musculocutaneous nerve, C5, 6.

Coracobrachialis

At: From the coracoid process of the scapula to the shaft of the humerus (medial border, half way down).
Ac: Flexion and adduction of the arm.
Ne: Musculocutaneous nerve, C5–7.

Brachialis

At: From the lower half of the front of the humerus to the tuberosity of the ulna (coronoid process).
Ac: Flexion of the forearm.
Ne: Musculocutaneous, C5, 6.

Triceps brachii

At: From the infraglenoid tubercle of the scapula (long head) and the posterior surface of the shaft of the humerus (lateral and medial heads) to the posterior surface of the olecranon of the ulna.
Ac: Extension of the forearm.
Ne: Radial nerve, C6–8.

Forearm muscles

Anterior superficial group of muscles

Pronator teres

At: From the common flexor origin (medial epicondyle of humerus) (humeral head) and coronoid process of ulna (ulnar head) to the middle of the lateral surface of the radius.
Ac: Pronation and flexion of the forearm.
Ne: Median nerve, C6, 7.

Flexor carpi radialis

At: From the common flexor origin to the bases of the second and third metacarpals.
Ac: Flexion and abduction of the wrist, flexion and pronation of the forearm.
Ne: Median nerve, C6, 7.

Palmaris longus

At: From the common flexor origin to the distal part of the flexor retinaculum.
Ac: Flexion of the wrist.
Ne: Median nerve, C7, 8.

Flexor carpi ulnaris

At: From the common flexor origin (humeral head) and posterior border of the ulna (ulnar head) to the pisiform bone and through it to the pisohamate and pisometacarpal ligaments.
Ac: Flexion and adduction of the wrist.
Ne: Ulnar nerve, C7, 8.

Flexor digitorum superficialis

At: From the common flexor origin and coronoid process of the ulna (humero-ulnar head) and the oblique line on the anterior surface of the radius (radial head) to the sides of the middle phalanges of the fingers.
Ac: Flexion of the wrist, metacarpophalangeal (MP) and proximal interphalangeal (IP) joints.
Ne: Median nerve, C7, 8, T1.

Anterior deep group of muscles

Flexor pollicis longus

At: From the anterior surface of the radius and interosseous membrane to the distal phalanx of the thumb.
Ac: Flexion of the thumb joints and wrist.
Ne: Median (anterior interosseous) nerve, C8, T1.

Flexor digitorum profundus

At: From the anterior and medial surfaces and posterior border of the ulna and interosseous membrane to the distal phalanx of the fingers.
Ac: Flexion of the finger joints and wrist.
Ne: Ulnar and median (anterior interosseous) nerves, C8, T1.

Pronator quadratus

At: From the lower anterior surface of the ulna to the lower anterior surface of the radius.
Ac: Pronation of the forearm.
Ne: Median (anterior inerosseous) nerve, C8, T1.

Posterior superficial group of muscles

Brachioradialis

At: From the lateral supracondylar ridge of the humerus to the radius above the styloid process.
Ac: Flexion and partial pronation of the forearm.
Ne: Radial nerve, C5, 6.

Extensor carpi radialis longus

At: From the lateral supracondylar ridge of the humerus to the base of the second metacarpal.
Ac: Extension and abduction of the wrist.
Ne: Radial nerve, C6, 7.

Extensor carpi radialis brevis

At: From the common extensor origin (lateral epicondyle of humerus) to the bases of the second and third metacarpals.
Ac: Extension and abduction of the wrist.
Ne: Radial nerve, C7, 8.

Extensor digitorum

At: From the common extensor origin to the dorsal digital expansions of the fingers.
Ac: Extension of the wrist and MP joints.
Ne: Radial nerve, C7, 8.

Extensor digiti minimi

At: From the common extensor origin to the dorsal digital expansion of the little finger.
Ac: Extension of the wrist and little finger.
Ne: Radial nerve, C7, 8.

Extensor carpi ulnaris

At: From the common extensor origin and posterior border of the ulna to the tubercle of the base of the fifth metacarpal.
Ac: Extension and adduction of the wrist.
Ne: Radial nerve, C7, 8.

Anconeus

> At: From the posterior surface of the lateral epicondyle to the olecranon and upper posterior surface of the ulna.
> Ac: Extension of the forearm.
> Ne: Radial nerve, C7, 8.

Posterior deep group of muscles

Supinator

> At: From the lateral epicondyle of the humerus, lateral and annular ligaments of the elbow joint and supinator crest of the ulna to the upper lateral third of the radius.
> Ac: Supination of the forearm.
> Ne: Radial nerve (posterior interosseous), C5, 6.

Abductor pollicis longus

> At: From the upper posterior surfaces of the radius and ulna and interosseous membrane to the base of the first metacarpal and trapezium.
> Ac: Abduction and extension of the thumb metacarpal.
> Ne: Radial nerve (posterior interosseous), C7, 8.

Extensor pollicis brevis

> At: From the posterior surface of the radius and interosseous membrane below the abductor to the base of the proximal phalanx of the thumb.
> Ac: Extension of the thumb, flexion and abduction of the wrist.
> Ne: Radial nerve (posterior interosseous), C7, 8.

Extensor pollicis longus

> At: From the middle part of the posterior surface of the ulna and interosseous membrane to the ulnar side of the dorsal digital expansion of the index finger.
> Ac: Extension of the index finger and wrist.
> Ne: Radial nerve (posterior interosseous), C7, 8.

Extensor indicis

> At: From the lower part of posterior surface of the ulna and interosseous membrane to the ulnar side of the dorsal digital expansion of the index finger.
> Ac: Extension of the index finger and wrist.
> Ne: Radial nerve (posterior interosseous), C7, 8.

Hand muscles

Adductor pollicis

> At: From the capitates, bases of second and third metacarpals and shaft of the third metacarpal to the ulnar side of the base of the proximal phalanx of the thumb.
> Ac: Adduction and opposition of the thumb.
> Ne: Ulnar nerve, C8, T1.

Lumbricals (4)

> At: From the tendons of flexor digitorum profundus in the palm to the radial sides of the dorsal digital expansions of the fingers.
> Ac: Flexion of MP joints and extension of IP joints of the fingers (with interossei).
> Ne: Median nerve (lateral two) and ulnar nerve (medial two), C8, T1.

Dorsal interossei (4)

> At: From the shafts of adjacent metacarpals to the dorsal digital expansions and bases of the proximal phalanges (2 and 3 to the radial and ulnar side of the middle finger, 1 to the radial side of the index finger, and 4 to the ulnar side of the ring finger).

Ac: Flexion of MP joints and extension of IP joints of the fingers (with lumbricals and palmar interossei); abduction of the fingers from baseline through the middle finger.
Ne: Ulnar nerve, C8, T1.

Thenar muscles
Abductor pollicis brevis
At: From the flexor retinaculum, trapezium and scaphoid to the radial side of the base of the first phalanx of the thumb.
Ac: Abduction and opposition of the thumb.
Ne: Median nerve, C8, T1.

Opponens pollicis
At: From the flexor retinaculum and trapezium to the anterior surface of the shaft of the first metacarpal.
Ac: Opposition of the thumb.
Ne: Median nerve, C8, T1.

Flexor pollicis brevis
At: From the flexor retinaculum and trapezium to the radial border of the proximal phalanx of the thumb.
Ac: Flexion and opposition of the thumb.
Ne: Median or ulnar nerve or both, C8, T1.

Hypothenar muscles
Palmaris brevis
At: From the palmar aponeurosis to the skin of the ulnar side of the hypothenar eminence.
Ac: Wrinkles the skin of the ulnar side of the palm.
Ne: Ulnar nerve, C8, T1.

Abductor digiti minimi
At: From the pisiform and piso-hamate ligament to the ulnar side of the base of the proximal phalanx and dorsal digital expansion of the little finger.
Ac: Abduction of the little finger.
Ne: Ulnar nerve, C8, T1.

Opponens digiti minimi
At: From the flexor retinaculum and hook of hamate to the ulnar border of the fifth metacarpal.
Ac: 'Cupping' of the hand.
Ne: Ulnar nerve, C8, T1.

Flexor digiti minimi brevis
At: From the flexor retinaculum and hook of hamate to the ulnar side of the base of the proximal phalanx of the little finger.
Ac: Flexion of the MP joint of the little finger.
Ne: Ulnar nerve, C8, T1.

TRUNK

Suboccipital muscles of the neck
Rectus capitis posterior major and minor
Obliquus capitis superior and inferior

Deep muscles of the back

Splenius capitis
At: From the spines of upper T vertebrae and lower ligamentum nuchae to the superior nuchal line and mastoid process.
Ac: Extension and rotation of the head.
Ne: Posterior rami of C3, 4.

Erector spinae
At: Spinalis (medial part), longissimus (intermediate part) and iliocostalis (lateral part), with multiple attachments to the vertebrae and adjacent parts of the ribs.
Ac: Extension of the spine and maintenance of posture.
Ne: Posterior rami of spinal nerves.

Transversospinales (semispinalis, multifidus, rotatores)

Interspinales and intertransversarii

THORAX

Diaphragm
At: **Lumbar part** from the crura (right, bodies of (LII–LIII) vertebrae and discs; left, bodies of L1 and L2 vertebrae and discs) and medial and lateral arcuate ligaments; **costal part** from the lower six costal cartilages and adjacent ribs; **sternal part** from the back of the xiphoid process; all converging to the central tendon, which has no bony attachment.
Ac: Inspiration, abdominal straining.
Ne: Phrenic nerve, C3–5.

Intercostals
At: **External**: downwards and forwards between adjacent ribs; **internal**: downwards and backwards between adjacent ribs; **innermost intercostals and subcostals** spanning more than one rib in lateral and some posterior parts of the thoracic cage.
Ac: Approximation of the ribs.
Ne: Intercostal nerves.

Transversus thoracis
At: From the body of the sternum to costal cartilages 2–6.
Ac: Approximation of the ribs.
Ne: Intercostal nerves.

Levatores costarum
At: From the transverse processes of (CVII–TXI) vertebrae to the rib below.
Ac: Elevation of the ribs.
Ne: Posterior rami of spinal nerves.

Muscles of the back

Serratus posterior superior
At: From the spines of (CVI–TII) vertebrae to ribs 2–5.
Ac: Elevation of the upper ribs.
Ne: Intercostal nerves.

Serratus posterior inferior
At: From the spines of (TXI–LII) vertebrae to the lowest four ribs.
Ac: Depression of the lower ribs.
Ne: Intercostal nerves.

ABDOMEN

Anterolateral muscles

Rectus abdominis

At: From the pubic crest, and body of pubis of the opposite side, to costal cartilages 5–7.
Ac: Flexion of the trunk, compression of the abdomen.
Ne: Intercostal nerves T7–12.

External oblique

At: From the lower eight ribs to the aponeurosis, fusing with the front of the rectus sheath and (lowest part) iliac crest, also forming the inguinal and lacunar ligaments.
Ac: Compression of the abdomen, depressioin of the ribs and flexion of the trunk.
Ne: Intercostal nerves T7–12.

Internal oblique

At: From the lateral part of the inguinal ligament, iliac crest and lumbar fascia to the lower four ribs, aponeurosis, which splits to form the rectus sheath and (lowest fibres) conjoint tendon.
Ac: Compression of the abdomen, depression of the ribs and flexion of the trunk.
Ne: Intercostal nerves T7–12, and iliohypogastric and ilioinguinal nerves, L1.

Transversus abdominis

At: From the lateral part of the inguinal ligament, iliac crest and lumbar fascia to the lower six costal cartilages, aponeurosis fusing with the back of the rectus sheath, and (lowest fibres) conjoint tendon.
Ac: Compression of the abdomen, depression of the ribs and flexion of the trunk.
Ne: Inguinal nerves, L1.

Cremaster (male)

At: From the internal oblique and transversus, spiralling down over the spermatic cord and returning to the internal oblique and pubic tubercle.
Ac: Retraction of the testes.
Ne: Genital branch of the genitofemoral nerve, L2.

Posterior muscles of the lower limb

Iliacus

At: From the iliac fossa to the tendon of psoas major and lesser trochanter of femur.
Ac: Flexion of the thigh and (acting from below) flexion of the trunk.
Ne: Femoral nerve, L2, 3.

Psoas major

At: From the sides of the lumbar vertebrae and intervertebral discs to the lesser trochanter of the femur.
Ac: Flexion of the thigh and (acting from below) flexion of the trunk.
Ne: L1–3.

Psoas minor

At: From the sides of T12 and L1 vertebrae to the iliopubic eminence.
Ac: Flexion of the lumbar spine.
Ne: Nerve from L1.

Quadratus lumborum

At: From the iliolumbar ligament and adjacent iliac crest to the medial part of the twelfth rib and transverse processes of L1–L4 vertebrae.
Ac: Stabilization and depression of the twelfth rib and lateral flexion of the lumbar spine.
Ne: Nerves from T12 and L1–4.

PELVIS

Lower limb muscles

Piriformis – see page 190, under Gluteal region

Obturator internus

Pelvic floor muscles

Levator ani

> At: From the pelvic surface of the body of the pubis and anterior part of the obturator fascia (pubococcygeus, forming puborectalis and levator prostatae [male] or pubovaginalis [female]) to the central perineal tendon and anococcygeal ligament, and the posterior part of the obturator fascia and inner surface of the ischial spine (iliococcygeus part) to anococcygeal body and coccyx.
> Ac: Pelvic floor, with puborectalis maintaining rectal continence.
> Ne: Perineal branches of S3, 4.

Coccygeus

> At: From the ischial spine and sacrospinous ligament to the coccyx and lowest part of the sacrum.
> Ac: Part of the pelvic floor.
> Ne: Perineal branches of S4, 5.

Perineal muscles

External anal sphincter

> At: From the tip of the coccyx to the central perineal tendon, with the upper part blending with the puborectalis part of the levator ani, and the lower part subcutaneous, curving inwards below the internal sphincter (smooth muscle).
> Ac: Maintenance of rectal continence.
> Ne: Inferior rectal branch of pudendal nerve, S3, 4.

Sphincter urethrae

> At: (Male) fibres encircle the membranous urethra within the deep perineal pouch and extend round the lower prostatic urethra, with some attachment to the pubic rami; (Female) fibres encircle the urethra.
> Ac: Sphincteric action on the urethra (external urethral sphincter).
> Ne: Perineal branch of the pudendal nerve, S3, 4.

Bulbospongiosus

> At: The central perineal tendon and perineal membrane to the midline raphe (male) or clitoris (female).
> Ac: Expulsion of urine and semen from the urethra (male) or constriction of the vaginal orifice (female).
> Ne: Perineal branch of the pudendal nerve, S3, 4.

Superficial transverse perineal muscles

Ischiocavernosus

Deep transverse perineal muscle (male)

LOWER LIMB

Gluteal region

Gluteus maximus

> At: From the posterior gluteal line of the hip bone, back of sacrum and sacrotuberous ligament to the iliotibial tract and gluteal tuberosity of the femur.

Ac: Extension and lateral rotation of the femur.
Ne: Inferior gluteal nerve, L5, S1, 2.

Gluteus medius

At: From the ilium between the anterior and posterior gluteal lines to the greater trochanter of the femur.
Ac: Abduction and medial rotation of the femur, and prevention of adduction.
Ne: Superior gluteal nerve, L4, 5, S1.

Piriformis

At: From the middle three segments of the sacrum to the greater trochanter of the femur.
Ac: Abduction and lateral rotation of the femur.
Ne: Nerves from L5, S1, 2.

Quadratus femoris

At: From the ischial tuberosity to the intertrochanteric crest of the femur.
Ac: Lateral rotation of the femur.
Ne: Own nerve, L5, S1, 2.

Obturator internus

At: From the inner surface of the obturator membrane to the greater trochanter of the femur.
Ac: Lateral rotation of the femur.
Ne: Own nerve, L5, S1, 2.

Gemellus superior and inferior

At: From the ischial spine and upper part of the ischial tuberosity, respectively, to the upper and lower
parts of the obturator internus.
Ac: Assists obturator internus.
Ne: Nerves to the obturator internus and quadrates femoris, respectively.

Obturator externus

At: From the outer surface of the obturator membrane and adjacent rami of the pubis and ischium to
the trochanteric fossa of the femur.
Ac: Lateral rotation of the thigh.
Ne: Obturator nerve, L3, 4.

Front of thigh muscles

Psoas major – see page 188, under **Posterior muscles of the lower limb**

Iliacus

Tensor fasciae latae

At: From the anterior part of the iliac crest to the iliotibial tract.
Ac: Extension and lateral rotation of the leg.
Ne: Superior gluteal nerve, L4, 5, S1.

Sartorius

At: From the anterior superior iliac spine to the upper medial surface of the shaft of the tibia in front of
the gracilis and semitendinosus.
Ac: Flexion, abduction and lateral rotation of the thigh.
Ne: Femoral nerve, L2, 3.

Rectus femoris

At: From the anterior inferior iliac spine (straight head) and ilium above the rim of the acetabulum to
the base of the patella.

Ac: Flexion of thigh and extension of the leg.
Ne: Femoral nerve, L3, 4.

Vastus lateralis

At: From the upper part of the intertrochanteric line, front of greater trochanter, gluteal tuberosity and upper linea aspera of the femur to the quadriceps tendon and patella.
Ac: Extension of the leg.
Ne: Femoral nerve, L2–4.

Vastus medialis

At: From the lower part of the intertrochanteric line, spiral line, linea aspera and medial supracondylar line of the femur to the quadriceps tendon and patella.
Ac: Extension of the leg.
Ne: Femoral nerve, L2–4.

Vastus intermedius

At: From the anterior and lateral parts of the upper two-thirds of the shaft of the femur to the deep part of the quadriceps tendon.
Ac: Extension of the leg.
Ne: Femoral nerve, L2–4.

Articularis genu

At: From the lower anterior surface of the shaft of the femur to the synovial membrane of the knee joint.
Ac: Retraction of the synovial membrane.
Ne: Femoral nerve, L2, 3.

Medial side of thigh muscles

Pectineus

At: From the pectineal line of the pubis to the femur between the lesser trochanter and linea aspera.
Ac: Flexion, adduction and lateral rotation of the thigh.
Ne: Obturator nerve, L2, 3.

Gracilis

At: From the body of the pubis and ischiopubic ramus to the upper medial surface of the shaft of the femur between the sartorius and semitendinosus.
Ac: Flexion, adduction and medial rotation of the thigh.
Ne: Obturator nerve, L2, 3.

Adductor brevis

At: From the body and inferior ramus of the pubis to the shaft of the femur between the lesser trochanter and upper linea aspera.
Ac: Adduction of the thigh.
Ne: Obturator nerve, L2–4.

Adductor longus

At: From the front of the pubis to the middle of the linea aspera of the femur.
Ac: Adduction of the thigh.
Ne: Obturator nerve, L2–4.

Adductor magnus

At: From the lower lateral part of the ischial tuberosity and ischiopubic ramus to the linea aspera of the femur and from the gluteal tuberosity down to the medial supracondylar line and adductor tubercle.

Ac: Adduction and lateral rotation of the thigh.

Ne: Obturator nerve, L2–4 and sciatic nerve, L4, 5, S1.

Back of thigh muscles

Biceps femoris

At: From the medial facet of the ischial tuberosity (longhead) and from the linea aspera and lateral supracondylar line of the femur (short head) to the head of the fibula.

Ac: Flexion and lateral rotation of the knee, and extension of the hip.

Ne: Sciatic nerve, L5, S1.

Semitendinosus

At: From the medial facet of the ischial tuberosity (with the long head of biceps) to the upper part of the subcutaneous surface of the tibia, behind the gracilis.

Ac: Flexion and medial rotation of the knee, and extension of the hip.

Ne: Sciatic nerve, L5, S1.

Semimembranosus

At: From the lateral facet of the ischial tuberosity to the groove on the back of the medial condyle of the tibia, with expansions forming the oblique popliteal ligament and fascia over the popliteus.

Ac: Flexion and medial rotation of the knee, and extension of the knee.

Ne: Sciatic nerve, L5, S1.

Front of leg and dorsum of foot muscles

Tibialis anterior

At: From the upper two-thirds of the lateral surface of the tibia and interosseous membrane to the medial surface of the medial cuneiform and base of the first metatarsal.

Ac: Dorsiflexion and inversion of the foot.

Ne: Deep fibular nerve, L4, 5.

Extensor hallucis longus

At: From the middle third of the medial surface of the fibula to the base of the distal phalanx of the great toe.

Ac: Extension of the great toe and dorsiflexion of the foot.

Ne: Deep fibular nerve, L5, S1.

Extensor digitorum longus

At: From the upper two-thirds of the medial surface of the fibula to the middle and distal phalanges of the lateral four toes.

Ac: Extension of the toes and dorsiflexion of the foot.

Ne: Deep fibular nerve, L5, S1.

Fibularis tertius

At: From the lower third of the medial surface of the fibula to the shaft of the fifth metatarsal.

Ac: Dorsiflexion and eversion of the foot.

Ne: Deep fibular nerve, L5, S1.

Extensor digitorum brevis

At: From the upper surface of the calcaneus to the tendons of the extensor hallucis longus and lateral three tendons of the extensor digitorum longus.

Ac: Extension of the toes.

Ne: Deep fibular nerve, L5, S1.

Lateral side of leg muscles

Fibularis longus

At: From the upper two-thirds of the lateral surface of the fibula to the lateral side of the medial cuneiform and base of the first metatarsal.
Ac: Plantarflexion and eversion of the foot.
Ne: Superficial fibular nerve, L5, S1, 2.

Fibularis brevis

At: From the lower two-thirds of the lateral surface of the fibula to the tuberosity of the base of the fifth metatarsal.
Ac: Plantarflexion and eversion of the foot.
Ne: Deep fibular nerve, L5, S1.

Back of leg and sole of foot muscles

Gastrocnemius

At: From the upper posterior part of the medial condyle of the femur (medial head) and lateral surface of the lateral condyle (lateral head) to the middle of the posterior surface of the calcaneus (by tendo-calcaneus [Achilles' tendon] with soleus).
Ac: Plantarflexion of the foot and flexion of the leg.
Ne: Tibial nerve, S1, 2.

Soleus

At: From the soleal line of the tibia, upper medial border of the tibia and upper posterior surface of the fibula to tendo-calcaneus (Achilles' tendon).
Ac: Plantarflexion of the foot.
Ne: Tibial nerve, S1, 2.

Plantaris

At: From the lateral supracondylar line of the femur to the medial side of the tendo-calcaneus (Achilles' tendon).
Ac: Plantarflexion of foot and flexion of the leg.
Ne: Tibial nerve, S1, 2.

Popliteus

At: From the back of the tibia above the soleal line to the outer surface of the lateral epicondyle of the femur.
Ac: Lateral rotation of the femur on fixed tibia (or *vice versa*).
Ne: Tibial nerve, L4, 5, S1.

Tibialis posterior

At: From the posterior surface of the interosseous membrane and adjacent surfaces of the tibia and fibula to the tuberosity of the navicular, with slips to other tarsal bones (except the talus) and middle metatarsals.
Ac: Plantarflexion and inversion of the foot.
Ne: Tibial nerve, L4, 5.

Flexor hallucis longus

At: From the lower two-thirds of the posterior surface of the fibula to the base of the distal phalanx of the great toe.
Ac: Plantarflexion of the great toe and foot.
Ne: Tibial nerve, S2, 3.

Flexor digitorum longus

At: From the medial part of the posterior surface of the tibia below the soleal line to the base of the distal phalanges of the four lateral toes.

Ac: Plantarflexion of the four lateral toes and foot.

Ne: Tibial nerve, S2, 3.

Sole of foot muscles – first layer

Abductor hallucis

At: From the medial process of the calcanean tuberosity and plantar aponeurosis to the medial side of the proximal phalanx of the great toe.

Ac: Abduction and plantar flexion of the great toe.

Ne: Medial plantar nerve, S2, 3.

Flexor digitorum brevis

At: From the medial process of the calcanean tuberosity and plantar aponeurosis to the sides of the middle phalanges of the four lateral toes, splitting to allow the tendons of flexor digitorum longus to pass through.

Ac: Plantarflexion of the toes.

Ne: Medial plantar nerve, S2, 3.

Abductor digiti minimi

At: From the lateral and medial processes of the calcanean tuberosity and plantar aponeurosis to the lateral side of the base of the proximal phalanx of the little toe.

Ac: Abduction and plantarflexion of the little toe.

Ne: Lateral plantar nerve, S2, 3.

Sole of foot muscles – second layer

Quadratus plantae

At: From the medial and plantar surfaces of the calcaneus to the lateral side of the flexor digitorum longus before it divides into tendons.

Ac: Assists plantarflexion of the four lateral toes.

Ne: Lateral plantar nerve, S2, 3.

Lumbricals

At: From the tendons of flexor digitorum longus to the medial sides of the dorsal digital expansions.

Ac: Plantarflexion of the four lateral MP joints and extension of IP joints (with interossei).

Ne: Medial plantar nerve (first lumbrical) and lateral plantar nerve, S2, 3.

Tendons of flexor digitorum longus and flexor hallucis longus

Sole of foot muscles – third layer

Flexor hallucis brevis

At: From the plantar surface of the cuboid and lateral cuneiform to both sides of the proximal phalanx of the great toe.

Ac: Plantarflexion of the MP joint of the great toe.

Ne: Medial plantar nerve, S2, 3.

Adductor hallucis

At: From the bases of the second, third and fourth metatarsals (oblique head) and plantar MP ligaments of the three lateral toes (transverse head) to the lateral side of the base of the proximal phalanx of the great toe (with part of the flexor hallucis brevis).

Ac: Adduction of the great toe.

Ne: Lateral plantar nerve, S2, 3.

Flexor digiti minimi brevis

At: From the plantar surface of the base of the fifth metatarsal to the lateral side of the base of the proximal phalanx of the little toe (with abductor digiti minimi).

Ac: Plantarflexion of the MP joint of the little toe.

Ne: Lateral plantar nerve, S2, 3.

Sole of foot muscles – fourth layer

Dorsal interossei (4)

At: From the adjacent sides of the shafts of the metatarsals to the bases of the proximal phalanges and dorsal digital expansions (1 and 2 to either side of the second toe, 3 and 4 to the lateral sides of the third and fourth toes).

Ac: Plantarflexion of the MP joints and extension of IP joints of the second, third and fourth toes (with lumbricals and plantar interossei); abduction of the toes from the second toe axis.

Ne: Lateral plantar nerve, S2, 3.

Plantar interossei (3)

At: From the bases of the medial sides of the third, fourth and fifth metatarsals to the medial sides of the bases of the proximal phalanges of the corresponding toe.

Ac: Plantarflexion of the MP joints and extension of IP joints of the three lateral toes (with dorsal interossei and lumbricals); adduction of the toes towards the second toe.

Ne: Lateral plantar nerve, S2, 3.

Tendons of fibularis longus and tibialis posterior

CRANIAL NERVES

For descriptive terms by long tradition, the twelve cranial nerves are identified by Roman numerals I–XII (1–12) within the cranial cavity and close to their foraminal entry/exit point.

I	Olfactory	VII	Facial
II	Optic	VIII	Vestibulocochlear
III	Oculomotor	IX	Glossopharyngeal
IV	Trochlear	X	Vagus
V	Trigeminal	XI	Accessory
VI	Abducent	XII	Hypoglossal

Principle function (PF); Cranial location (CL); Origin and cranial course (OCC):

I OLFACTORY NERVE

PF: Smell – special sensory.
CL: Anterior cranial fossa – cribriform plate of the ethmoid bone.
OCC:
- From the submucosa of the olfactory epithelium of the upper nasal cavity through the roof of the nose.
- Fine nerve filaments (about 20 in number) ensheathed in dura mater pass through the multiple foramina in the cribriform plate of the ethmoid bone into the anterior cranial fossa to reach and enter the under surface of the olfactory bulb at the distal end of the olfactory tract.

II OPTIC NERVE

PF: Vision – special sensory
CL: Middle cranial fossa – optic canal (within the sphenoid between the body and two roots of the lesser wing).
OCC:
- From the retina of the eye, a single large nerve which is approximately 4 cm in total length.
- It passes posteromedially back through the orbital cavity and the optic canal to unite with the optic chiasma on the base of the brain.

III OCULOMOTOR NERVE

PF: Motor/parasympathetic:
- To four muscles that move the eye (superior rectus, inferior rectus, medial rectus and inferior oblique).
- Also to levator palpebrae superioris, which elevates the upper eyelid.
- The nerve also contains parasympathetic fibres that constrict the pupil and alter the curvature of the lens
CL: Middle cranial fossa – superior orbital fissure (within the sphenoid between the body and the greater and lesser wings, with a portion of the frontal bone at the lateral extremity).
OCC:
- Emerges from the medial side of the cerebral peduncle sometimes as several rootlets that quickly merge into one nerve.

- The nerve passes forwards, downwards and laterally and pierces the dura mater to enter the roof of the cavernous sinus high in the lateral wall, from which it descends and at the anterior end divides into a superior and inferior branch.
- Both nerve branches pass into and through the superior orbital fissure to enter the orbital cavity.

IV TROCHLEAR NERVE

PF: Motor – to one of the eye muscles (superior oblique) that depresses and laterally rotates the eye.

CL: Middle cranial fossa – superior orbital fissure (within the sphenoid between the body and the greater and lesser wings, with a portion of frontal bone at the lateral extremity).

OCC:

- Single and thin-strand-like, it is the only cranial nerve to emerge from the dorsal surface of the brain-stem (from the midbrain behind the inferior colliculus).
- From here it crosses to the lateral side of the superior cerebellar peduncle, turns around the side of the cerebral peduncle above the pons and passes forwards onto the free edge of the tentorium cerebelli which it runs along for a short distance then pierces it to enter the cavernous sinus.
- It then traverses along the lateral wall of the sinus and passes into and through the superior orbital fissure to enter the orbital cavity.

V TRIGEMINAL NERVE

PF: Sensory/motor – the main sensory nerve of the head, which includes, the face and surface of the eye; and motor nerve to the masticatory muscles (for chewing) and jaw movement.

CL: Middle cranial fossa – apex of the petrous part of the temporal bone.

OCC:

- The largest of the cranial nerves it emerges as a large (sensory) and smaller (motor) root from the ventral surface of the pons close to its upper border.
- Together the nerves pass forwards and angle over the petrous part of the temporal bone beneath the dura mater covering the floor of the anterior cranial fossa.
- They then descend to join the trigeminal ganglion within the trigeminal cave (which is formed by the trigeminal depression in the temporal bone).
- From the trigeminal ganglion stem three main nerve divisions:
  - (V1) Ophthalmic nerve – exits the superior orbital fissure to enter the orbital cavity.
  - (V2) Maxillary nerve – exits the foramen rotundum in the greater wing of the sphenoid.
  - (V3) Mandibular nerve – exits the foramen ovale at the base of the skull.

VI ABDUCENT NERVE

PF: Motor – to one of the eye muscles (lateral rectus) that rotates the eye laterally.

CL: Middle cranial fossa – superior orbital fissure (within the sphenoid between the body and greater and lesser wings, with a portion of frontal bone at the lateral extremity).

OCC:

- Emerges as a single nerve from the brainstem near the midline at the junction of the pons and the pyramid of the medulla.
- It passes forwards slightly upwards and laterally through the cisterna pontis to pierce the dura mater covering the clivus just below and lateral to the dorsum sellae of the sphenoid.
- It continues upwards beneath the dura mater and then bends forwards over the tip of the petrous part of the temporal bone beneath the petrosphenoidal ligament to enter and pass through the body of the cavernous sinus.
- It then passes through the superior orbital fissure to enter the orbital cavity.

VII FACIAL NERVE

PF: Motor/sensory/parasympathetic: to the muscles of the face, and containing some taste fibres and parasympathetic lacrimal, salivary and nasal glands.

CL: Posterior cranial fossa – internal acoustic meatus (in the posterior surface of the petrous part of the temporal bone).

OCC:

- Emerges from the lateral cerebellopontine angle as a (sensory) root, the nervous intermedius, and a (motor) root along with the vestibulocochlear nerve.
- The sensory root, the nervous intermedius, is situated between the facial and vestibulocochlear nerves, hence its name.
- The nerve roots run antero-laterally to enter the internal acoustic meatus and continue laterally in the facial canal above the vestibule of the inner ear, where they unite to form a single nerve.
- The nerve runs on to reach the genicular ganglion (in the medial wall of the epitympanic recess) and then makes a right-angle turn backwards in the medial wall of the middle ear (above the promontory) and passes downwards in the medial wall of the aditus to the mastoid antrum.
- It then exits the stylomastoid foramen in the base of the skull.

VIII VESTIBULOCOCHLEAR NERVE

PF: Motor/sensory: combined nerve for balance (the vestibular part) and hearing (the cochlear part).

CL: Posterior cranial fossa – internal acoustic meatus.

OCC:

- Emerges from the lateral cerebellopontine angle (along with the two roots of the facial nerve).
- It runs antero-laterally to enter the internal acoustic meatus where it divides into the vestibular and cochlear nerves.
- The vestibular nerve divides into upper and lower branches, the upper branch goes on to supply the semi-circular canals and utricle whilst the lower branch supplies the saccule.
- The cochlear nerve enters the temporal bone in the antero-inferior quadrant and goes to the cochlear modiolus.

IX GLOSSOPHARYNGEAL NERVE

PF: Sensory/parasympathetic: some taste fibres, and other sensory fibres for the lining of the throat, and a small but important percentage of parasympathetic fibres for reflex control of blood pressure.

CL: Posterior cranial fossa – jugular foramen (between the jugular fossa of the petrous, temporal and occipital bones).

OCC:

- Emerges as three or four rootlets from the side of the brainstem lateral to the olive of the medulla oblongata along with the vagus and cranial part of the accessory nerve.
- The rootlets quickly merge and form into one nerve that passes forwards antero-laterally and enters the jugular foramen, which it exits at the base of the skull.

X VAGUS NERVE

PF: Motor/sensory/parasympathetic: to larynx, pharynx and soft palate (for speech and swallowing), gastric secretion and movement, and slowing the heart rate. Afferent from many thoracic and abdominal viscera.

CL: Posterior cranial fossa – jugular foramen (between the jugular fossa of the petrous part of the temporal and occipital bones).

OCC:

- Emerges as eight or ten rootlets from the side of the brainstem lateral to the olive of the medulla oblongata along with the glossopharyngeal and cranial part of the accessory nerve.
- The rootlets merge to form a single nerve that passes forwards into and through the jugular foramen at the base of the skull.

XI ACCESSORY NERVE

PF: The spinal part goes to the sternocleidomastoid and trapezius, with other fibres (the cranial part) joining the vagus nerve to supply the larynx, pharynx and soft palate.

CL: Posterior cranial fossa – jugular foramen (between the jugular fossa of the petrous part of the temporal and occipital bones).

OCC:

- The accessory nerve has a (**cranial root**) and a (**spinal root**).
- The **cranial root** emerges as four or five rootlets from the side of the brainstem lateral to the olive of the medulla oblongata along with the glossopharyngeal and vagus nerves.
- These rootlets form into a single nerve that travels antero-laterally a short distance before being joined by the single spinal root.
- The **spinal root** emerges as a series of rootlets from the lateral side of the upper five or six cervical segments of the spinal cord dorsal to the denticulate ligament.
- These rootlets unite to form a single nerve that runs up the side of, and parallel to, the medulla oblongata to join the cranial nerve root.
- Together both **cranial** and **spinal** nerve roots pass forwards into and through the jugular foramen in the base of the skull.

XII HYPOGLOSSAL

PF: Motor: to tongue muscles.

CL: Posterior cranial fossa – hypoglossal canal (in the occipital bone above the anterior part of the condyle).

OCC:

- Emerges from the medulla oblongata between the pyramid and the olive as a series of 10–15 rootlets that merge and form two nerves; these pass posterior to the vertebral artery and enter the hypoglossal canal where they unite and exit as a single nerve at the base of the skull.

GLOSSARY OF ANATOMICAL TERMS

Many words used in medical practice today, and in particular descriptive terms for anatomical structures, derive in the main from Latin (L) and Greek (G). This short selective Glossary provides the opportunity to gain a clearer understanding of some of the terminology in current use.

A

abdomen – L
  probably meaning to hide
abduct – L
  to draw out from the midline
abducent – L
  leading from
acetabulum – L
  little vinegar cup
acoustic – G
  related to hearing
acromion – G
  extremity of shoulder
adenoid – L
  gland-like
aditus – L
  opening or entrance
adrenal – L
  towards the kidney
afferent – L
  carrying to
ala – L
  a wing
alba – L
  white
alveolus – L
  a hollow, small space
ampulla – L
  globular flask
anastomosis – G
  towards a mouth; joining together
annulus – L
  ring
ansa – L
  handle or loop
anteversion – L
  forward turn
antrum – L
  cave

anus – L or Anglo Saxon
  to sit
aorta – G
  to lift or heave
aponeurosis – G
  derived from a sinew
appendix – L
  appendage
aqueduct – L
  to lead water
arachnoid – G
  spider-like
areola – L
  courtyard or little open space
artery – G
  keeping air (arteries were thought to contain air)
articulation – L
  a joint
arytenoid – G
  like a ladle
atlas – G
  Greek god, bearing the earth on his shoulders
atrium – L
  court or hall
auricle – L
  ear
axilla – L
  armpit
axis – G
  an axle, to carry
azygos – G
  unpaired, not yoked

B

basilic – G
  important or prominent
biceps – L
  two heads

brachium – L
  arm
brevis – L
  short
bronchus – G
  windpipe
buccal – L
  cheek
buccinator – L
  trumpeter
bulla – L
  large vesicle
bursa – L
  purse

C

caecum – L
  blind
calcaneus – L
  heel
calcarine – L
  spur-shaped
callosum – L
  thick
calyx – G
  a cup
canaliculus – L
  little canal
canine – L
  dog-like
canthus – G
  niche or corner
capitate – L
  head-like
capitulum – L
  little head
capsule – L
  a box or case
cardiac – G and L
  heart
carina – L
  keel of a boat
carotid – G
  heavy sleep (from the Greek belief that the carotid arteries caused drowsiness)
carpus – G and L
  wrist
caudate – L
  tail

cavernous – L
  full of cavities
cephalic – G
  head
cerebellum – L
  little brain
cerebrum – L
  brain
cervix – L
  neck
chiasma – G
  crossed lines, like the Greek letter chi
choana – G and L
  funnel
chondro – G
  cartilage
chorion – G
  skin or leather used as a membrane
choroid – G
  like a vascular membrane
cilia – L
  eyelashes
circumflex – L
  bending
clavicle – L
  little key
clitoris – G
  shut up
clivus – L
  slope
cloaca – L
  sewer
coccyx – G
  cuckoo, whose beak the bone resembles
cochlea – L
  snail or snail shell
coeliac – G and L
  belly
colliculus – L
  little hill
colon – G and L
  large intestine
commitans – L
  an accompanying person
communicans – L
  share with someone, connecting or joining

concha – L
  shell
condyle – L
  joint or knuckle
conjunctiva – L
  join together
conoid – G
  cone-like
coracoid – G
  crow-like, beak like a crow's
cornea – L
  horn
coronary – L
  encircling like a crown
corpus – L
  body
cortex – L
  bark or shell
cornu – L
  a horn
cranium – G and L
  upper part of head
cremaster – G
  a suspender
cribriform – L
  sieve-like
cricoid – G
  ring-like
crista – L
  a crest
cruciate – L
  crossed
cruciform – L
  cross-shaped
crus – L
  shin
crura – L
  legs
cubital – L
  elbow
cuneate, cuneiform – L
  wedge-shaped
cusp – L
  pointed-tip
cutaneous – L
  skin
cyst – G and L
sac or bladder

D

dartos – G
  skinned or flayed
decussation – G
  crossing like the letter x
deferens – L
  carrying away
deltoid – G
  triangular like the uppercase fourth letter
  of the Greek alphabet
dens – L
  tooth
dermatome – G
  cutting skin
dermis – G
  skin
diaphragm – G
  through a fence, a partition
diastole – G
  a pause, a place apart, expansion
digastric – G
  double belly
digit – L
  finger or toe
diploe – G
  double
dorsum – L
  back
duct – L
  to lead
duodenum – L
  twelve (length of twelve fingerbreadths)
dura mater – L
  tough mother

E

ectopic – G
  out of place
efferent – L
  carrying out
ejaculation – L
  throwing out
embryo – G
  to swell
endocrine – G
  to secrete inside
endolymph – G
  water inside

enteric – G
  intestine
epidermis – G
  upon the skin
epididymis – G
  upon the testicle
epigastrium – G
  upon the belly or stomach
epiglottis – G
  upon the tongue
epiphysis – G
  growing upon or extra growth
epiploic – G
  floating
epithelium – G
  upon the nipple
erythrocyte – G
  red cell
ethmoid – G
  sieve-like
extensor – L
  stretch out

F

falciform – L
  sickle-shaped
fascia – L
  bandage or sash
fauces – L
  passage
femur – L
  thigh
fenestra – L
  window, opening
fibula – L
  buckle or brooch
filiform – L
  thread or hair-like
fimbria – L
  fringe or border
fissure – L
  cleft or groove
flexion – L
  bending
foetus – L
  to bring forth, offspring
follicle – L
  leather ball or money bag

fontenelle – L
  little spring or fountain
foramen – L
  small opening
fornix – L
  arch
fossa – L
  ditch
fovea – L
  small pit
frenulum – L
  bridle or curb
frontal – L
  forehead or brow
fundus – L
  bottom of a cavity

G

galea – L
  helmet made of leather
galli – L
  cock
ganglion – G
  knot or swelling
gastric – G
  stomach
gastrocnemius – G
  stomach of the leg
gemellus – L
  twin, paired
genitalia – L
  reproductive organs belonging to birth
genu – L
  knee
gingiva – L
  gum
glabella – L
  smooth, hairless
glans – L
  acorn
glenoid – G
  socket-like
glomerulus – L
  little ball
glottis – G
  vocal apparatus
gluteus – L
  rump

gomphosis – G
  nail
gonad – G
  seed
gracile – L
  slender
gyrus – G and L ring or circle

H

hallux – L
  great toe
hamate – L
  hooked
haustrum – L
  machine for drawing water
hemi – G
  half
hepatic – G
  liver
hernia – L
  protrusion through an opening
hiatus – L
  gape
hilum – L
  small bit, trifle
hormone – G
  to excite
humerus – L
  shoulder
humour – G
  liquid
hyaline – G
  glassy
hydro – G
  water
hymen – G
  membrane
hyoid – G
  U-shaped, from the Greek letter u
hyper – G
  above, in excess of
hypo – G
  under, deficient
hypophysis – G
  undergrowth
hypothenar – G
  under the palm
hyster – G
  uterus

I

ileum – G and L
  small intestine, twisting
ilium – L
  loin
ima – L
  lowest
incisor – L
  cut into
incus – L
  an anvil
index – L
  forefinger, point out
infra – L
  below or under
infundibulum – L
  funnel
inguinal – L
  groin
inion – G
  back of the head
innominate – L
  without a name
insula – L
  island
iris - G and L
  rainbow
ischium – G an L
  hip
isthmus – G
  narrow passage or entrance

J

jejunum – L
  empty, hungry
jugular – L
  neck, throat or collar bone

K

keratin – G
  horn
kyphosis – G
  bent or bowed

L

labium, labrum – L
  lip
labryrinth – G
  maze

lacerum – L
  jagged
lacrimal – L
  tear
lactation – L
  milk
lacuna – L
  pit or hollow, pool or pond
lamina – L
  plate or layer
larynx – G
  upper windpipe
lateral – L
  side or flank
latissimus – L
  widest
leminiscus – G and L
  ribbon
leucocyte – G
  white cell
levator – L
  lifter
ligament – G
  to bind or tie
ligature – L
  bond or tie
linea – L
  linen thread
lincal – L
  spleen, splenic
lingual – L
  tongue
lordosis – G
  bend the body forwards
lumbar – L
  loin
lumbrical – L
  earthworm
lunate – L
  crescent-shaped
lutea – L
  yellow
lymph – L
  clear water

M

macula – L
  small spot, mark
magnus – L

  great
malleolus – L
  little hammer
malleus – L
  hammer
mamillary – L
  nipple
mamma – L
  breast
mandible – L
  lower jaw, chew
manubrium – L
  handle
manus – L
  hand
masseter – G
  chewer
mastoid – G
  breast-like
maxilla – L
  jawbone
maximus – L
  biggest
meatus – L
  passage
medial – L
  towards the midline
median – L
  in the midline
mediastinum – L
  median partition
medius – L
  middle
medulla – L
  marrow
meninges – G
  membranes
meniscus – G and L
  crescent
mental – L
  chin
mesentery – G
  middle intestine
mesoderm – G
  middle skin
metacarpus – G
  after wrist
metopic – G

between eyes

micturition – L
  desire to pass urine

minimus – L
  smallest

mitral – L
  Bishop's cap

molar – L
  mill for grinding

morphology – G
  study of form or shape

motor – L
  mover

myenteric – G
  intestinal muscle

myocardium – G
  heart muscle

N

nares – L
  nostril

navicular – L
  small boat

nephron – G
  kidney

neuron – G
  nerve or sinew

node – L
  knot

nucleus – L
  kernel, small nut

O

obturator – L
  plug an opening

occiput – L
  back of the head

oculomotor – L
  eye mover

ocular – L
  eye

odontoid – G
  tooth-like

oesophagus – G
  carrying food

olecranon – G
  head of the elbow

olfactory – G
  make smell

omentum – L
  fatty

omos – G
  shoulder

ophthalmic – G
  eye

opponens – L
  placing against

optic – G and L
  sight

oral – L
  mouth

orbit – L
  track or circuit

os – L
  mouth (plural ora)

os – L
  bone (plural ossa)

ossification – L
  make bone

ostium – L
  door or opening

otic – G
  pertaining to the ear

ovary – L
  receptacle for egg

ovum – L
  egg

P

palate – L
  palate

palpebra – L
  eyelid

pampiniform – L
  tendril-shaped

pancreas – G
  all flesh

papilla – L
  nipple

para – G
  beside

paralysis – G
  loosen alongside

parietal – L
  wall

parotid – G
  near the ear

patella – L
  flat dish
pectinate – L
  like a comb
pectoral – L
  breast
pedicle – L
  little foot
peduncle – L
  stalk
pelvis – L
  basin
penis – L
  tail
peri – G
  around, about
perilymph – G
  water around
perineum – G
  evacuate around
periodontal – G
  around tooth
peripheral – G
  carry around
peritoneum – G
  stretch around
peroneal – G
  brooch
pes – I
  foot
petrous – G
  stony
phalanx – G
  line of soldiers
pharynx – G
  throat
philtrum – L
  love charm
phrenic – G
  mind or heart as centre of emotions
pia mater – L
  soft mother
pineal – L
  pine cone
piriform – L
  pear-shaped
pituitary – L
  mucus (the gland was thought to secrete
  mucus)

placenta – L
  cake
plantar – L
  sole of foot
platysma – G
  broad
pleura – G
  rib, side
plexus – L
  network
plica – L
  fold
pollex – L
  thumb
pons – L
  bridge
popliteus – L
  ham
porta – L
  entrance
prepuce – L
  foreskin
profundus – L
  deep
pronation – L
  bend forwards
proprioceptive – L
  take one's own
prostate – G
  stand before
psoas – G
  loin muscle
pterion – G
  wing
pterygoid – G
  wing-like
ptosis – G
  falling
pubis – L
  secondary sex hair
pudendal – L
  ashamed
pulmonary – L
  lung
punctum – L
  sharp point
pupil – L
  doll (from image reflected in cornea)

pylorus – G
  gatekeeper

Q

quadrate – L
  four-sided

quadriceps – L
  four-headed

R

radius – L
  spoke

ramus – L
  branch

raphe – G
  seam

rectus – L
  straight

recurrent – L
  run back

renal – L
  kidney

retina – L
  net

retinaculum – L
  hold back, retain

retro – L
  behind or backwards

rima – L
  cleft

rotundum – L
  round

ruga – L
  wrinkle or crease

S

saccule – L
  small sac or pouch

sagittal – L
  arrow

salpinx – G
  tube, trumpet

saphenous – G
  apparent, not hidden

sartorius – L
  tailor (sitting cross-legged)

scala – L
  staircase

scalene – G
  triangle with unequal sides

scaphoid – G
  boat-shaped

scapula – L
  shoulderblade

sciatic – G
  hip

sclera – G
  hard

scrotum – L
  bag

sebaceous – L
  grease

sella – L
  saddle

semen – L
  seed

seminiferous – L
  carrying seed

serratus – L
  toothed

sesamoid – G
  like a sesame seed

sigmoid – G
  like the letter s

sinus – L
  curve or hollow

skeleton – G
  dried up

spermatozoa – G
  seed animals

sphenoid – G
  wedge-like

sphincter – G
  tight binder

splanchnic – G
  organ

squamous – L
  scale-like

stapes – L
  stirrup

sternum – G and L
  breast, breast bone

striation – L
  furrowed by lines

stroma – G
  bed, framework

styloid – G
  pillar-like

sulcus – L
  groove
supination – L
  bend backwards
sural – L
  calf
sustentaculum – L
  to hold up, support
suture – L
  seam
sympathetic – G
  with feeling
symphysis – G
  growing together
synovial – G
  with egg (like white of egg)
systole – G
  contraction, draw together

T

taenia – G
  fillet, tape or band
talus – L
  ankle
tarsus – G
  flat surface
tectum – L
  cover or roof
temporal – L
  time (temples, where hair first goes grey)
tentorium – L
  tent
tegmen – L
  covering
tendon – G
  stretch out
teres – L
  round and long
testicle – L
  diminutive of testis
thalamus – G
  chamber, bedroom
thenar – G
  palm of hand
thorax – G and L
  breastplate
thrombus – G
  curd, clot

thymus – G
  sweetbread (like a bunch of thyme flowers)
thyroid – G
  shield-like
tibia – L
  flute
trabecula – L
  little beam
trachea – G
  rough air channel
tragus – G
  goat (goat-like like hairs in front of the ear)
triceps – G
  three-headed
triquetral – L
  three-cornered
trochanter – G and L
  runner
trochlea – G and L
  pulley
tuber – L
  protuberance
turbinate – L
  child's top
tympanum – G and L
  drum

U

ulna – L
  elbow
umbilicus – L
  navel
uncinate – L
  hooked
ureter – G and L
  urinary canal
uterus – L
  leather water bottle
uvula – L
  little grape

V

vagina – L
  sheath
vagus – L
  wandering
vallecula – L
  little hollow

vas deferens – L
  vessel carrying away
ventral – L
  toward the belly side
ventricle – L
  little belly
vermiform – L
  worm-like
vertebra – L
  turning joint
vesicle – L
  little bladder
viscus – L
  internal organ
vestibule – L
  space between the entrance and street

volar – L
  palm of hand or sole of foot
vomer – L
  ploughshare
vulva – L
  wrapper

X
xiphoid – G
  sword-like

Z
zona – G
  belt, girdle or zone
zygomatic – G
  yoke

BIBLIOGRAPHY

MAIN REFERENCE

Gray's Anatomy, 40th edn. S. Standring (ed). Churchill Livingstone, 2008.

TERMINOLOGY

Terminologia Anatomia. Federative Committee on Anatomical Terminology. Thieme, 1998.

Anatomical Eponyms. Jessie Dobson. E & S Livingstone Ltd., 1962.

A Dictionary of Scientific Terms. I.F. Henderson, W.D. Henderson. Oliver & Boyd, 1920.

LEGAL AND HISTORICAL REFERENCE

The Disposal of the Dead. C.J. Polson, T.K. Marshall. English Universities Press, 1975.

DISSECTION GUIDES

Dissection Guide for Human Anatomy. D.A. Morton, K.D. Peterson, K.H. Albertine. Churchill Livingstone, 2004.

ILLUSTRATED ATLASES

Gray's Anatomy for Students, 3rd edn. R.L. Drake, A.W. Vogl, A.W.M. Mitchell. Churchill Livingstone, 2015.

McMinn & Abrahams' Clinical Atlas of Human Anatomy, 7th edn. P.H. Abrahams, J.D. Spratt, M. Loukas, A.N. Van Schoor. Elsevier-Mosby, 2013.

McMinn's Colour Atlas of Foot and Ankle Anatomy, 4th edn. B.M. Logan, R.T. Hutchings. Elsevier–Saunders: 2012.

Atlas of Human Anatomy, 5th edn. F.H. Netter. Saunders–Elsevier, 2011.

A Colour Atlas of Anatomy, 7th edn. J.W. Rohen, C. Yokochi, E. Lutjen-Drecoll. Schattauer–Lippincott Williams & Wilkins, 2011.

McMinn's Colour Atlas of Head and Neck Anatomy, 4th edn. B.M. Logan, P.A. Reynolds, R.T. Hutchings. Mosby–Elsevier, 2010.

Grant's Atlas of Anatomy, 12th edn. A.M. Agur, A.F. Dalley. Lippincott Williams & Wilkins, 2009.

Human Anatomy Color Atlas, 5th edn. J.A. Gosling, P.F. Harris, J.R. Humpherson, I. Whitmore, P.L.T. Whillan. Mosby–Elsevier, 2008.

Anatomy a Regional Atlas of the Human Body, 5th edn. C.D. Clemente. Lippincott Williams & Wilkins, 2007.

A Colour Atlas of Applied Anatomy. R.M.H. McMinn, R.T. Hutchings, B.M. Logan. Wolfe Medical Publications, 1984.

ILLUSTRATED TEXT BOOKS

Essential Clinical Anatomy, 5th edn. K.L. Moore, A.M. Agur, A.F. Dalley. Wolters Kluwer, 2015.

Clinical Anatomy by Regions, 9th edn. R. Snell. Wolters Kluer–Lippincott Williams & Wilkins, 2012.

Clinical Anatomy, 12th edn. H. Ellis, V. Mahadevan. Wiley–Blackwell, 2006.

Principles of Human Anatomy, 10th edn. G.J. Tortora. J. Wiley, 2005.

McMinn's Functional and Clinical Anatomy. R.M.H. McMinn, P. Gaddum-Rosse, R.T. Hutchings, B.M. Logan. Mosby, 1995.

Last's Anatomy Regional and Applied, 9th edn. R.M.H. McMinn, Churchill Livingstone, 1994.

Textbook of Anatomy. A.W. Rogers. Churchill Livingstone, 1992.

Cranial Nerves. L. Wison-Pauwels, E.J. Akeson, P.A. Stewart. B.C. Decker, 1988.

Anatomy of Orofacial Structures. R.W. Brand, D.E. Isselhard. Mosby, 1977.

Anatomy Regional and Applied, 4th edn. R.J. Last. J. & A. Churchill, 1970.

QUICK REFERENCE

Anatomy at a Glance, 3rd edn. O. Faiz, S. Blackburn, D. Moffat. Wiley–Blackwell, 2011.

Human Sectional Anatomy Pocket Atlas, 3rd edn. H. Ellis, B.M. Logan, A.K. Dixon. Hodder Arnold, 2009.

Crash Course – Anatomy, 3rd edn. M. Dykes, W. Watson. Mosby–Elsevier, 2007.

Instant Anatomy, 3rd edn. R.H. Whitaker, N.R. Borley. Blackwell Science, 2005.

Clinical Anatomy, a Core Text with Self Assesment, S. Monkhouse. Churchill Livingstone, 2001.

The Concise Handbook of Human Anatomy. R.M.H. McMinn, R.T. Hutchings, B.M. Logan. Manson Publishing, 1998.

RADIOLOGY/IMAGING/ANATOMY

Human Sectional Anatomy, 4th edn. H. Ellis, B.M. Logan, A.K. Dixon, D.J. Bowden. Taylor & Francis CRC Press, 2015.

Imaging Atlas of Human Anatomy, 4th edn. J. Weir, P.H. Abrahams, J.D. Spratt, L.R. Salkowski. Mosby–Elsevier, 2011.

Anatomy for Diagnostic Imaging. S. Ryan, M. McNicholas, S. Eustace. Saunders, 2004.

SURFACE ANATOMY

Surface Anatomy, 4th edn. J.S.P. Lumley. Churchill Livingstone, 2008.

Clinical Surface Anatomy. K.M. Backhouse, R.T. Hutchings. Mosby Year Book, 1998.

A Concise Colour Guide to Clinical Surface Anatomy. N.R. Borley. Manson Publishing, 1997.

ANATOMICAL AND PREPARATION TECHNIQUES

Biological Museum Methods, Vol. 1 & 2. G. Hangay, M. Dingley. Academic Press, 1985.

Digging Up Bones, 3rd edn. D.R. Brothwell. Oxford University Press, 1981.

Mortuary Science. F.C. Gale. C.C. Thomas, 1981.

Techniques in Biological Preparation. J. Simpkins. Blackie, 1974.

Anatomical Techniques, 2nd edn. D.H. Tompsett. E. & S. Livingstone, 1970.

The Preservation of Natural History Specimens, Vol. 1 Invertebrates, Vol. 2 Vertebrates, Botany, Geology. R. Wagstaffe, J.H. Fiddler. Witherby, 1968–1970.

Anatomical Preparations. M. Hildebrand. University of California Press, 1968.

Teaching and Display Techniques in Anatomy and Zoology. T.F. Spence. Pergamon Press, 1967.

Medical Museum Technology. J.J. Edwards, M.J. Edwards. Oxford University Press, 1959.

Artistic and Scientific Taxidermy and Modelling. M. Browne. A. & C. Black, 1896 (extensive bibliography on techniques).

The Practical Naturalists' Guide. J.B. Davies. Maclachlan & Stewart, 1858.

The Anatomical Instructor. T. Pole. Couchman & Fry, 1790.

Index

Index

Note: Page references in *italic* refer to boxed text